P9-API-742

## Cooking Well

# Thyroid Health

## Marie-Annick Courtier

### Foreword by Lauren Feder, M.D.

*Cooking Well: Thyroid Health*

Text copyright © 2010 Marie-Annick Courtier

All rights reserved. No part of this book may be reproduced, stored in a retrieval system, or transmitted, in any form or by any means, electronic or otherwise, without written permission from the Publisher.

Hatherleigh Press is committed to preserving and protecting the natural resources of the Earth. Environmentally responsible and sustainable practices are embraced within the company's mission statement. Hatherleigh Press is a member of the Publishers Earth Alliance, committed to preserving and protecting the natural resources of the planet while developing a sustainable business model for the book publishing industry.

This book was edited and designed in the village of Hobart, New York. Hobart is a community that has embraced books and publishing as a component of its livelihood. There are several unique bookstores in the village. For more information, please visit www.hobartbookvillage.com.

www.hatherleighpress.com

DISCLAIMER
This book offers general cooking and eating suggestions for educational purposes only. In no case should it be a substitute nor replace a healthcare professional. Consult your healthcare professional to determine which foods are safe for you and to establish the right diet for your personal nutritional needs.

Library of Congress Cataloging-in-Publication Data

Courtier, Marie-Annick.
  Cooking well. Thyroid health / Marie-Annick Courtier ; foreword by Lauren Feder.
    p. cm.
  Includes bibliographical references.
  ISBN 978-1-57826-352-3 (pbk. : alk. paper) 1. Thyroid gland--Diseases--Popular works. 2. Thyroid gland--Diseases--Diet therapy--Recipes. 3. Cookbooks. I. Title. II. Title: Thyroid health.
  RC655.C66 2010
  641.5'631--dc22
                              2010032872

All Hatherleigh Press titles are available for bulk purchase, special promotions, and premiums. For information about reselling and special purchase opportunities, please call 1-800-528-2550 and ask for the Special Sales Manager.

Cover Design by Nick Macagnone
Cover Photography by Catarina Astrom
Interior Design by Nick Macagnone
10 9 8 7 6 5 4 3 2 1

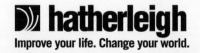

**hatherleigh**
Improve your life. Change your world.

# Table of Contents

# Acknowledgments

Hatherleigh Press would like to extend a special thank you to Jo Brielyn—without your hard work and dedication this book would not have been possible.

# Foreword

After reading *Cooking Well: Thyroid Health*, I feel that the concept of utilizing nutrition to improve thyroid health has now received its well-deserved place in health and wellness books. Thyroid conditions are being diagnosed in epidemic proportions, and millions of Americans must now rely on daily medication to treat these disorders. Because of this, there is a tremendous need to consider additional options to support healthy thyroid function.

Thyroid health is a personal matter for me as I underwent two surgeries for hyperthyroidism as a teenager. During my medical residency 10 years later, I consulted with a holistic practitioner at a friend's recommendation. He treated my remaining thyroid gland with natural medications and diet. Within a short period of time I was able to discontinue my medications and I have never needed any treatment since.

The important role of the thyroid cannot be overstated, as it affects a myriad of functions throughout the body. Medical advancements in the 20th century have been impressive in their achievements and more sophisticated techniques, including complex drugs and antibiotics, have saved many lives and improved quality of health. However, many people are concerned about side-effects from thyroid medication. Dissatisfied with a lifetime prescription of medication, many are interested in learning about additional ways to improve thyroid health.

Most patients and their physicians consider a diagnosis of a thyroid condition—whether it be hypothyroidism or hyperthyroidism—as a lifelong regimen of daily medication. Yet the concept of health is multi-faceted and *Cooking Well: Thyroid Health* brings to light additional options available to a person diagnosed with a thyroid condition. Although some people may always require medication, food can be a wonderful medicine. Hippocrates wrote, "Let food be your medicine and medicine be your food". More and more doctors are recognizing the significant role that nutrition plays in general health, including thyroid health.

The recipes in this book are appealing to the contemporary palate while also being therapeutic by design. These delicious recipes of healthy food choices were chosen specifically to regulate thyroid function whether you have hypothyroidism or hyperthyroidism.

Beginning with the descriptive facts of both hypothyroidism and hyperthyroidism, the book provides a well-rounded balance of easy-to-understand science and excellent recipes. Whether you are a novice in the kitchen or a gourmet chef, these recipes are both delicious and simple to prepare. Readers will be delighted with the practical applications and how-to recipes to be used for thyroid health. People who are conscientious about health will also find the suggested "Foods to Avoid and Foods to Choose" section sensible and easy to follow. This book has greatly expanded my opportunity as a physician to counsel my patients regarding diet and thyroid health.

—*Lauren Feder, M.D.*

# Chapter 1

# Understanding Thyroid Health

**The thyroid gland is a small, yet vital member of the endocrine system.** The butterfly-shaped organ, which sits at the front of the neck and directly below the larynx, provides hormones to the entire body. Its hormones, thyroxine (T4) and triiodothyronine (T3), function to regulate metabolism, body temperature, and growth and development. T3 and T4 also control the rate at which the body's cells perform their duties, so disease that prevents the thyroid gland from working properly inevitably throws the entire body out of balance.

According to the third U.S. National Health and Nutritional Examination Survey conducted by the Centers for Disease Control and Prevention (CDC), over 12.2 million Americans, almost 6% of the population, are reported to have thyroid disease. Eighty percent of those individuals, roughly 9.6 million, live with *hypothyroidism* (underactive thyroid). The other 2.6 million have *hyperthyroidism* (overactive thyroid). Since thyroid disease affects the body so diversely and may create symptoms often associated with other illnesses, it often goes undetected or undiagnosed for quite some time before a proper diagnosis is reached.

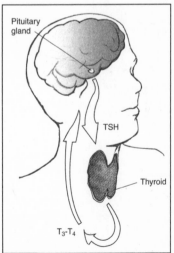

Image courtesy of the National Institute of Diabetes and Digestive and Kidney Disease.

Because this disease affects so many individuals, it is important to understand thyroid disease, recognize the symptoms of both conditions, and learn how the right diet can help improve the quality of life for those living with thyroid conditions. Both hypothyroidism and hyperthyroidism can generally be managed with medication and the proper diet, but a lifetime commitment to this balanced regimen is required in order for individuals who have thyroid disease to live a healthy, active life.

# Hypothyroidism

Hypothyroidism, also sometimes referred to as *myxedema*, is the more common of the two conditions. It occurs when the thyroid gland is underactive and fails to produce enough thyroid hormones (T3 and T4). Common causes of hypothyroidism are inflammation of the gland, which damages the cells (such as Hashimoto's thyroiditis, an autoimmune disorder in which the immune system attacks the thyroid gland); congenital birth defects; exposure to radioactive iodine; radiation treatments of the neck in cancer treatments; viral thyroiditis (inflammation of the thyroid gland, which can cause excess thyroid hormones to leak into the bloodstream); or surgical removal of a portion of the thyroid gland. In addition, women—especially those over the age of fifty—are more likely to develop this condition.

Hypothyroidism affects the growth, development and cellular processes throughout the body. If left untreated or not properly treated, the condition may lead to other disorders. Complications may include, but are not limited to, low blood sugar, heart disease, infertility, miscarriages, low blood sugar, and decreased breathing.

It is important to remember there is not yet a known cure for hypothyroidism. It is, however, possible to treat and manage it with a proper combination of medication and dietary

**Common Symptoms of Hypothyroidism:**
- Fatigue
- Constipation
- Joint and/or muscle pain
- Sensitivity to cold
- Pale or dry skin
- Anemia
- Difficulty losing weight
- Weakness
- Depression
- Heavier menstruation
- Thin or brittle hair and/or nails
- Weight gain

**Symptoms that may develop later include:**
- Slow speech
- Puffy face, hands, and feet
- Decreased senses of smell and taste
- Hoarseness
- Thickening of the skin

changes. In the majority of cases, hypothyroid patients are given daily doses of T4 (the thyroid hormone thyroxine) or levothyroxine sodium, a synthetic form of the thyroid hormone. An average daily dosage of T4 is about 100 to 150 micrograms. The medication is also known to reduce cholesterol levels in patients. Individuals who also have heart conditions should not receive this type of treatment and will need to seek alternative methods with their physicians.

Holistic approaches such as acupuncture, yoga, breathing exercises, and stress relief are also recommended for hypothyroidism patients because they relieve muscle aches and emotional problems (namely depression) associated with the condition.

In addition to taking daily dosages of thyroid hormone, individuals living with hypothyroidism must also incorporate a healthy diet into their lifestyle. One of the most effective changes for improving the health of hypothyroid patients is the increase of iodine-rich foods in their diets.

# Hyperthyroidism

An overactive thyroid, or hyperthyroidism, causes the gland to make an overabundance of thyroid hormones (T3 and T4). There are a number of illnesses and conditions which may cause hyperthyroidism to occur. Among them are Graves disease (an autoimmune disorder which causes antibodies in the immune system to attack the thyroid gland), noncancerous growths on the thyroid gland or pituitary gland, adenoma (occurs when part of the gland separates itself from the rest of the gland and forms benign tumors that may cause an overproduction of thyroid hormones) and toxic multinodular goiter (an enlarged thyroid gland which has small growths, or nodules, attached to it causing overproduction of T3 and T4 hormones), inflammation of the thyroid (thyroiditis) caused by viral infections, intake of excessive amounts of iodine, abnormal secretion of the thyroid-stimulating hormone (TSH or thyrotropin), an excessive intake of thyroid hormones, and tumors of the ovaries and testes.

When an individual has an excessive amount of thyroid hormones in his or her blood stream, it may also lead to a complication called *thyrotoxicosis,* or thyroid crisis. This is often caused by an infection or an increase in stress. Signs of thyrotoxicosis include fever, abdominal pain, and decreased mental alertness. Hospitalization is necessary to treat this complication.

There are two main antithyroid drugs generally prescribed to individuals with hyperthyroidism: propylthiouracil and methimazole. Both medications function to block the production of thyroid hormones. Another common therapy used for hyperthyroidism is radioactive iodine (RAI) which is given to patients as a capsule or dissolved in water. The stomach and intestines absorb it and carry it via the bloodstream to the thyroid gland. Once in the thyroid, the RAI interrupts the function of some of the thyroid cells and slows down the overproduction of T3 and T4 hormones.

In addition to medical treatments, there are numerous holistic approaches that prove beneficial in improving the physical and mental wellbeing of individuals living with hyperthyroidism. These include methods such as yoga, acupuncture, stress relief and breathing exercises.

Patients with hyperthyroidism may find it more difficult to gain weight, so they are often put on a high-calorie diet. The most effective foods for improving symptoms include those high in healthy calories, but not high in fat. Individuals should add more liquids (water, milk, and juices) to their regimen to avoid constipation and diarrhea, two symptoms often associated with hyperthyroidism. They are also encouraged to increase their consumption of vitamins A, B, C, and E through dietary changes and supplements.

**Common Symptoms of Hyperthyroidism:**
- Heat intolerance
- Rapid heart rate
- Weight loss
- Excessive sweating
- Tremors or shaking
- Fatigue
- Increased bowl movements
- Decreased concentration
- Nervousness or agitation
- Difficulty sleeping
- Enlarged thyroid gland at the base of the neck (goiter)
- Irregular or scant menstrual flow

**Symptoms that may develop later include:**
- Heart problems (rapid heart rate, heart rhythm disorders, congestive heart failure)
- Brittle bones or osteoporosis
- Blurring or double vision
- Redness and swelling of the skin (usually the legs and feet)

# How the Right Diet Can Help

## Hypothyroidism

For hypothyroidism patients, the key to enhancing thyroid function is adequate, but not excessive, iodine intake. The thyroid gland uses iodine to produce T3 and T4. Therefore, boosting the amount of iodine in the body will also increase the natural production of hormones and promote thyroid health. People with hypothyroidism generally have a deficiency in their iodine levels. A desirable iodine intake for the average person is in the range of 100 to 300 micrograms per day. To determine the recommended intake for treating hypothyroidism, patients should request an iodine test and a blood sample to measure their thyroid-related hormone levels.

Tyrosine, a nonessential amino acid, also helps improve the function of various organs responsible for making and regulating hormones, such as the thyroid, pituitary, and adrenal glands. Tyrosine is found in a variety of healthy food choices.

These and other helpful additions to the diet will be discussed in further detail in Chapter 2.

## Hyperthyroidism

When thyroid hormones are overactive, as they are for individuals with hyperthyroidism, more energy is used by the body. To balance this increased demand on the body and provide extra energy, high-calorie foods should be added to the diet.

To combat constipation, which is common among hyperthyroidism patients, a variety of high-fiber foods should also be incorporated into one's diet.

An increase in fluid intake is also helpful for those dealing with hyperthyroidism as this condition can often cause diarrhea, constipation, and dehydration. To avoid such complications, individuals should drink at least six to eight glasses of liquids (such as water, milk, and natural juices) daily.

These and other useful dietary suggestions will be covered in the next chapter.

# Chapter 2

# The Importance of Nutrition

## Dietary Suggestions for a Healthy Lifestyle

### Hypothyroidism

As discussed in the previous chapter, iodine is used by the thyroid gland to produce thyroid hormones. Individuals living with hypothyroidism generally have low iodine levels and should consider eating foods which are high in iodine. Iodine-rich foods include seafood, seaweed, sea salt, and whole-wheat bread. Other excellent sources of natural iodine—as well as important vitamins, minerals, and nutrients—that should be included are spinach, tomatoes, carrots, kelp, peas, radishes, mushrooms, potatoes, onions, squash, asparagus, strawberries, eggs, and low-fat yogurt. As a general rule, "ground-grown" foods (such as carrots, potatoes, squash, and beans) contain higher levels of iodine because they absorb it from the soil, so eating foods grown in the ground which contain healthy levels of iodine is most beneficial. Since chlorine found in regular tap water may deplete or interfere with iodine levels in the body, it is also recommended to switch to bottled or distilled water for drinking.

The amino acid tyrosine also helps with the health and function of the thyroid gland. Natural sources of tyrosine can be found in chicken, pumpkin seeds, lentils, almonds, turkey, avocado, bananas, sesame seeds, and fish.

Consuming foods high in protein and taking supplements of vitamins B and D are also healthy additions for those with hypothyroidism.

# Hyperthyroidism

For people living with hyperthyroidism, a high-calorie diet is key for maintaining a healthy energy level. Since overactive thyroid hormones cause the body to use more energy, increasing the consumption of calorie-rich foods will increase energy levels. Healthy, high-calorie choices include breads (whole-wheat, pumpernickel, rye, and oat bran); vegetables high in starch (potatoes, peas, winter squash, beets, carrots, and corn); healthy spreads (hummus, peanut butter, honey, jam, and low-fat cream cheese); fruits (bananas, pears, pineapple, and apples); cereals (granola and muesli); hearty soups (chili with beans, lentil, minestrone, black bean, and split pea soups); and dried fruits (peaches and dates).

Foods containing goitrogens, natural substances that slow down the production of thyroid hormones, are also beneficial for those with hyperthyroidism. Food sources include broccoli, Brussels sprouts, cabbage, kale, cauliflower, spinach, soybeans, pine nuts, and peanuts.

Items high in calcium also help relieve symptoms of hyperthyroidism. Choose non-fat and low-fat options such as reduced-fat milk, non-fat yogurt, cheese (Swiss, mozzarella, American, cottage, and Parmesan), frozen yogurt, beans (black, navy, and soy), green leafy vegetables, fortified cereals, almonds, tofu, and oysters.

High-fiber foods such as beans,

**Natural Sources of Vitamin B:**
- Meats
- Poultry
- Nuts
- Legumes
- Green vegetables
- Dairy
- Whole grains

**Natural Sources of Vitamin D:**
- Dairy products
- Eggs
- Tuna
- Cod
- Mackerel
- Sea bass
- Liver oils

**Natural Sources of Vitamin A:**
- Dairy
- Green leafy vegetables
- Yellow vegetables
- Liver
- Fruits

**Natural Sources of Vitamin C:**
- Citrus
- Berries
- Green vegetables
- Papayas

**Natural Sources of Vitamin E:**
- Vegetable oils
- Dark green leafy vegetables
- Nuts
- Wheat germ
- Whole grains

cereals, whole-grain breads and pastas, vegetables, fruits, and natural juices (such as prune juice) are recommended. In addition, eating foods high in zinc and taking supplements of vitamins A, C and E are recommended for those with hyperthyroidism.

# Foods to Avoid

### Hypothyroidism

Just as consuming the right foods can aid in thyroid health, eating the wrong foods can heighten symptoms of hypothyroidism. For individuals who have this condition, it is especially important to avoid foods which interfere with the body's ability to absorb iodine. Products such as white table salt and chlorine should be replaced with healthier choices like sea salt and bottled water. Avoid excessive amounts of turnips, garlic, white flour, pears, and peaches as these also hinder the absorption of iodine.

Foods rich in goitrogens (like broccoli, Brussels sprouts, cabbage, kale, cauliflower, spinach, soybeans, pine nuts, and peanuts), fluoride, and caffeine should also be limited in order to aid in thyroid function.

### Hyperthyroidism

Individuals with hyperthyroidism should steer clear of any foods that contain high amounts of iodine. The thyroid gland uses iodine to produce thyroid hormones, and people with hyperthyroidism already have an abundance of those hormones. Adding more iodine to the body will only lead to further complications. Items to avoid include iodized salt or sea salt, seafood, dairy products, eggs, plants grown in iodine-rich soil, and iodine supplements.

Smoking can aggravate or increase the production of thyroid hormones and should be ceased or, at the bare minimum, drastically decreased.

Consumption of foods and drinks containing caffeine should also be avoided or limited as these can add to the effects of hyperthyroidism, causing a more rapid heart rate, nervousness, and difficulty with concentration.

> **Note:** Any recipes that call for low-fat ingredients can be substituted with whole fat.

# Chapter 3

# The Recipes

The following sections contain recipes categorized by hypothyroidism and hyperthyroidism. Any recipes that are safe for both conditions have been marked for easy reference.

Because seafood contains high amounts of iodine, it is recommended that hyperthyroidism patients avoid any seafood dishes. See page 9 for more information.

Some of the following recipes call for garlic or salt. Be sure to adjust or eliminate these ingredients to suit your dietary needs. You can also try substituting salt with Mrs. Dash® salt-free seasonings.

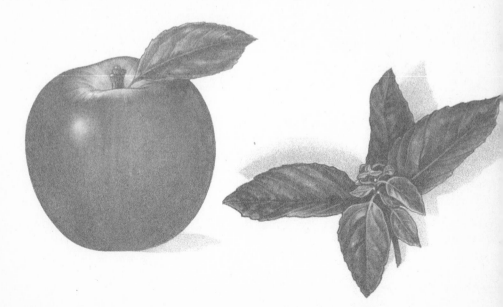

# Breakfast

## Hypothyroidism

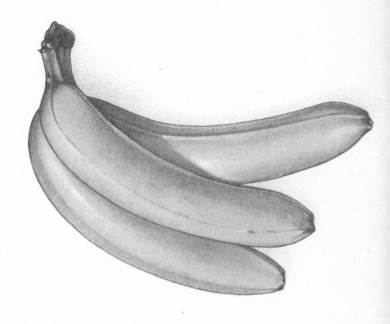

# Breakfast Smoothie

serves 2

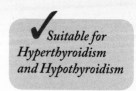

✓ *Suitable for Hyperthyroidism and Hypothyroidism*

## ingredients

4 ounces pure pomegranate juice, no sugar added
1 cup mixed berries
1 small banana
½ cup apple juice, no sugar added
1 tablespoon flaxseeds
Ice cubes

## cooking instructions

Place all the ingredients in a blender and fill with ice. Puree on high speed until smooth. Divide between two tall glasses and serve immediately with a straw.

# Cheese Blintzes with Raspberries

serves 4

## ingredients

*For the crêpes:*
1 cup sifted flour
2 extra-large eggs, beaten
1 tablespoon honey, warmed in
the microwave
2 tablespoons unsalted butter,
melted
Pinch salt

1 cup low-fat milk
2 cups fresh raspberries

*For the filling:*
1½ cups low-fat cottage cheese
¼ cup low-fat sour cream
1 tablespoon honey, warmed in
the microwave
Pinch salt

## cooking instructions

*For the filling:* Mix in a bowl the cottage cheese, sour cream, honey, and salt. Refrigerate until use.

Place 1 cup of the raspberries in a blender and reduce to a sauce. Pass through a sieve to remove seeds and refrigerate until use.

*For the crêpes:* Place the flour in a bowl. Blend in the eggs, honey, salt, and melted butter. Slowly whisk in the milk. Let the batter rest for 30 minutes. Before use, add a little water to thin out the batter.

Heat a nonstick pan or crêpe pan over medium heat. Soak a small piece of paper towel in vegetable oil and swirl quickly over the pan. Add enough batter and swirl to cover the entire bottom. Cook until golden brown and remove from heat. Do not cook the other side. Repeat until all the batter has been used.

Place the golden brown side of the crêpes side up. Divide the filling among the center length of the crêpes. Roll a bit, tuck both edges, and finish rolling to retain all the filling inside the crêpes. Cook the crêpes over medium heat in a greased skillet until golden brown on all sides. Serve immediately with the raspberry coulis and the remaining raspberries.

# French Toast with Orange Slices

serves 4

> ✓ *For variety you may flavor with cinnamon and nutmeg.*

## ingredients

3 eggs
⅔ cup low-fat milk
1½ teaspoons orange extract
Pinch salt
8 slices whole wheat bread
Vegetable oil
4 tablespoons maple syrup
2 oranges, peeled and sliced

## cooking instructions

Beat together the eggs, milk, orange extract, and salt. Dip the bread slices in the mixture. Soak them well.

Preheat two large skillets or a griddle with a little vegetable oil. Add the bread slices and brown on both sides. Serve immediately with maple syrup and orange slices.

# Granola with Banana, Apple, and Walnut

serves 2

## ingredients

½ cup granola
½ cup low-fat milk
¼ small banana, peeled and sliced
¼ medium apple, peeled, cored, and diced
1 teaspoon chopped walnuts

## cooking instructions

Mix the granola with the milk. Add the banana, apples, and walnuts, and serve immediately.

# Orange Wheat Muffins with Cream Cheese

**serves 12**

## ingredients

1 cup unbleached all-purpose flour

½ cup whole wheat flour

½ cup flaxseed meal

⅓ cup honey

1 teaspoon baking soda

1 tablespoon baking powder

¼ teaspoon salt

1 teaspoon orange extract

1 teaspoon orange zest

2 large eggs

2 tablespoons canola oil

½ cup pumpkin puree (organic can)

1 cup plain low-fat yogurt

12 tablespoons low-fat cream cheese

12 teaspoons pumpkin seeds

Pumpkin pie spices or cinnamon to taste (optional)

## cooking instructions

Preheat the oven to 375° F.

Blend the flours, flaxseed meal, honey, baking soda, baking powder, and salt in a mixing bowl. Blend in the orange extract, orange zest, canola oil, eggs, pumpkin puree, yogurt, and mix well. Fill muffin pan and bake for 25 minutes or until cooked through and golden brown.

Top each muffin with 1 tablespoon of low-fat cream cheese. Sprinkle spices or cinnamon, pumpkin seeds, and serve immediately.

# Rye Bread with Cream Cheese and Salmon

serves 1

✓ *Option: You may mix in a bit of freshly minced dill and some lemon juice into the cream cheese before spreading over the bread.*

## ingredients

1½ tablespoons low-fat cream cheese
1 slice rye bread
1 slice smoked salmon (about ¾ ounces)
Lemon juice

## cooking instructions

Spread the cream cheese over the bread. Add the smoked salmon, sprinkle a little lemon juice, and serve immediately.

# Scrambled Eggs with Mushrooms and Onions

serves 2

## ingredients

1 teaspoon olive oil
½ small yellow onion, chopped
(about 2 ounces)
4 white mushrooms, sliced
(about 4 ounces)

1 garlic clove, minced (optional)
1 tablespoon freshly minced basil
4 eggs
1 tablespoon low-fat milk
Salt and pepper to taste

## cooking instructions

Heat the oil in a nonstick pan over medium heat. Add the onion and sauté until translucent. Add the garlic, mushrooms, and sauté until mushrooms are cooked through. Beat the eggs with the milk in a bowl. Add the basil and season to taste. Pour the mixture over the vegetables. Cook over medium heat, stirring and scraping the bottom and sides of the pan constantly with a wooden spoon. As soon as the eggs begin to set, remove from heat, continue to stir for a few seconds, and serve immediately.

# Breakfast

## Hyperthyroidism

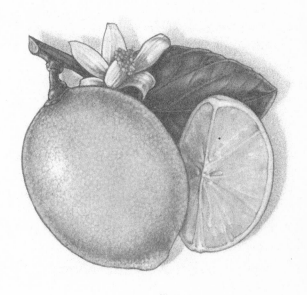

# Strawberry, Pomegranate, and Spinach Smoothie

✓ *This breakfast smoothie can also be used for a snack during the day.*

serves 2

## ingredients

2 cups strawberries
(about 10 ounces)
1 bunch fresh spinach
(at least 2 cups)
1 small banana

1 pomegranate
1 tablespoon flaxseeds
Ice cubes

## cooking instructions

De-seed the pomegranate. Place the seeds in a blender and add the remaining ingredients. Fill with ice and puree on high speed until smooth. Divide between two tall glasses and serve immediately with a straw.

# Cream of Millet

serves 1

## ingredients

1 cup low-fat rice or almond milk
Small pinch salt
1 teaspoon pumpkin pie spices
(optional)
¼ cup pearl millet
2 teaspoons slivered almonds
2 teaspoons maple syrup

½ peach, peeled, seeded,
and diced
1 teaspoon flaxseed oil

✔ *If you use less cooking liquid, the millet grain is fluffier and crunchier. Try it with ¾ cup of the soy milk instead of the 1 cup used in the recipe. Using more liquid creates a more moist, soft texture. This is all about personal preference, so experiment and find the texture you like.*

*Substitute the peach with apricot, apple, or mango.*

## cooking instructions

Warm the milk, salt, and pumpkin pie spices over medium heat in a small saucepan. Wash the millet a couple of times and drain well. Place the millet in another pan over medium heat. Add the almonds and the warm flavored milk. Reduce heat and simmer for 20 minutes or until all the liquid is absorbed.

Transfer to a serving bowl and mix in the maple syrup. Top with the fruits, drizzle flaxseed oil, and serve immediately.

# Homemade Granola

**serves 10**

## ingredients

¼ cup honey

¼ cup grapeseed oil

2 teaspoons cinnamon

1 teaspoon almond extract

1 teaspoon orange extract

3½ cups rolled oats

¼ cup slivered almonds

¼ cup chopped walnuts

## cooking instructions

Preheat the oven to 350°F. In a bowl, mix the honey, spices, oil, and extracts. Stir in the oats and nuts. Mix well and spread over a greased cookie sheet. Bake for 10 minutes. Stir and continue to bake for another 10 minutes, or until golden brown. Cool completely and break apart. Store in an airtight container away from heat.

You may substitute the honey with agave nectar. Enjoy with low-fat soy milk, low-fat rice milk, low-fat almond milk, low-fat milk, low-fat plain yogurt, or a mix of low-fat milk and low-fat plain yogurt. Top with your favorite fruits for added nutritional values.

Add 1 teaspoon freshly ground flaxseeds per serving before serving.

# Muesli with Dried Fruit and Nuts

serves 1

## ingredients

½ cup muesli cereal
½ cup low-fat rice or almond milk
1 tablespoon mixed dried berries
1 tablespoon raisins
1 teaspoon slivered or sliced almonds
1 teaspoon chopped walnuts

## cooking instructions

In a bowl, mix the cereal with the milk. If too thick, add a little more milk to thin out. Top with the mixed dried berries, raisins, almonds, and walnuts, and serve immediately.

# Oat Bran–Flax Muffin

serves 12

## ingredients

1 cup unbleached all-purpose flour
½ cup oat bran flour
½ cup flaxseed meal
½ cup brown sugar
1½ teaspoons baking soda
1 teaspoon baking powder
¼ teaspoon salt
1½ tablespoons ground cinnamon
1 teaspoon ground ginger
1¼ cups shredded peeled carrots

2 medium apples, peeled, cored, and finely diced
¾ cup walnuts, chopped
¾ cup dried berries and raisins blend (about equal amount of each)
¼ cup canola oil
1 teaspoon vanilla extract
2 eggs, mixed
½ cup rice or almond milk

✓ *Careful, this recipe can act as a laxative. It is advisable to eat only one muffin per day. Muffins can be frozen once individually wrapped in cellophane and then placed in a freezer bag. For best results, defrost at room temperature for 1 hour.*

## cooking instructions

Preheat the oven to 350°F.

In a bowl, blend the flours, flaxseed meal, brown sugar, baking soda, baking powder, salt, cinnamon, and ginger. Mix in the carrots, apples, walnuts, and berry-raisin blend. Add the oil, vanilla, eggs (or banana and apple sauce mixture), and milk, and mix until incorporated. Grease the muffin tin with canola oil. Divide mix among the 12 cups of a muffin tin and bake between 20 to 25 minutes.

You can substitute the eggs with equal parts mashed banana and apple sauce, equaling the same net weight as the eggs.

# Whole Grain Bread with Almond Butter, Pears, and Walnuts

serves 1

## ingredients

1 tablespoon almond butter
1 slice whole grain bread
½ medium pear, peeled, cored, and sliced
½ teaspoon chopped walnuts

## cooking instructions

Spread the almond butter over the bread. Layer the pear slices on top, sprinkle with walnuts, and serve immediately.

# Soups & Salads

## Hypothyroidism

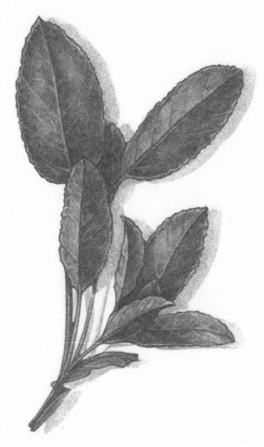

# Grapefruit and Crabmeat Salad

serves 2

## ingredients

1 large pink grapefruit
(about 16 ounces grapefruit)
8 ounces crabmeat portions,
excess water removed
2 tablespoons low-fat canola
mayonnaise

1 cup lettuce, shredded
1 tablespoon freshly minced
cilantro
Chili powder to taste
Salt and pepper to taste

## cooking instructions

Place the crabmeat in a bowl.

Cut the grapefruit in half. Insert a thin knife all around the skin to loosen up the flesh. Separate the flesh from the skin and place it on a cutting board. Dice the flesh small and transfer to the crabmeat bowl. Add mayonnaise, chili powder, cilantro, and season to taste. Cover with plastic wrap and refrigerate for half an hour.

Equally divide the lettuce in two plates and top with the prepared grapefruit crabmeat salad.

# Greek Salad with Cod

serves 4

## ingredients

4 tablespoons vinaigrette
1 teaspoon freshly minced oregano
4 cups mixed greens
1 large cucumber, peeled, seeded, and sliced (about 12 ounces)
2 large tomatoes, sliced (about 12 ounces)

½ small red onion, sliced (about 2 ounces)
1 medium red bell pepper, seeded, ribs removed, and sliced (about 6 ounces)
¼ cup black olives
4 tablespoons feta cheese
Four 4-ounce cooked cod fillets
Salt and pepper to taste

## cooking instructions

Mix the vinaigrette with the oregano and set aside.

Divide the mixed greens, cucumber, tomatoes, red onion, bell pepper, black olives, and feta cheese among 4 plates. Top with the fish fillet and season with salt and pepper. Drizzle with the vinaigrette and serve immediately.

# Smoked Salmon, Potato, and Watercress Salad

serves 4

## ingredients

12 ounces smoked salmon, diced
3 cooked potatoes, sliced (about 1 pound)
1 bunch watercress
1 cup cooked green beans
1 hardboiled egg, chopped (or 2 egg whites for less cholesterol)

2 tablespoons white wine vinegar
4 tablespoons olive oil
1 teaspoon Dijon mustard
1 tablespoon minced shallots
2 tablespoons minced salad herbs
Salt and pepper to taste

## cooking instructions

Mix the vinegar, mustard, and shallots in a bowl. Whisk in the olive oil, 1 tablespoon of minced herbs, and season to taste.

Mix half of the dressing with the potatoes. Mix the remaining dressing with the watercress. Divide the watercress among four plates. Top with the potatoes, broccoli, and salmon. Sprinkle with the chopped egg, remaining minced herbs, and serve immediately.

# Sugar Snap Peas and Tuna Salad

**serves 4**

## ingredients

*For the salad:*
4 ounces Boston lettuce
1½ cans tuna in water, strained (9 ounces)
1 large carrot, thinly sliced (about 4 ounces)
2 large tomatoes, seeded and diced
1 cup fresh sugar snap peas (about 4 ounces)
Salt and pepper to taste

*For the dressing:*
1 shallot, minced
1 garlic clove, minced (optional)
3 tablespoons lemon juice
3 tablespoons olive oil
2 tablespoons salad herbs
Salt and pepper to taste

## cooking instructions

Heat a steamer and add the sugar snap peas. Cook for 2 minutes. Add the carrots and continue to steam for 2 minutes or until desired doneness. In a bowl, mix the shallot, garlic, lemon juice, oil, 1 tablespoon of herbs, and season to taste. In a large bowl mix the lettuce with half of the dressing. Add the tuna, tomatoes, carrot slices, and sugar snap peas. Sprinkle with the remaining herbs and dressing before serving.

# Tomato, Mozzarella, and Basil Salad

serves 4

## ingredients

6 large tomatoes, sliced
(about 2¼ pounds)
1 shallot, minced
1 garlic clove, minced (optional)
4 tablespoons olive oil
2 tablespoons white wine or apple
cider vinegar

8 fresh basil leaves
8 ounces fresh mozzarella cheese,
sliced

## cooking instructions

Spread the tomatoes over a large platter. Sprinkle with salt and set aside for 20 minutes. Mince half the basil leaves and set aside. Shred the remaining leaves and set aside.

Mix the shallot, garlic, and vinegar in a bowl. Whisk in the oil, the minced basil, and season to taste.

Transfer the tomatoes to another serving platter. Alternate a tomato slice and mozzarella slice. Spread the shredded basil, pour the dressing over, and serve immediately.

# Carrot and Apple Soup

serves 4

## ingredients

5 large carrots, peeled and sliced (about 20 ounces)
1 large Golden Delicious apple, peeled and quartered (about 6 ounces)
1 medium onion, peeled and quartered (about 6 ounces)

4 cups gluten-free chicken stock (low-fat and low-sodium)
1 bouquet garni
¼ teaspoon ground ginger
Salt and pepper to taste

## cooking instructions

Place the carrots, apple, onion, stock, bouquet garni, and ginger in a large pan. Bring to boil over medium heat. Reduce heat, cover, and simmer until the vegetables are cooked through, 10 to 15 minutes. Transfer to a blender and puree with enough of the liquid to obtain a soup consistency. Season with salt and pepper and serve immediately.

# Cod and Corn Chowder

serves 4

## ingredients

2 teaspoons grapeseed oil

1 medium onion, diced (about 6 ounces)

1 medium carrot, diced (about 3 ounces)

1 large celery stalk, diced (about 2 ounces)

2 medium potatoes, peeled and diced (about 12 ounces)

Corn kernels from 2 corn ears

2 cups vegetable stock (low-fat and low-sodium)

1 cup low-fat milk

1 pound cod fish fillets, diced

2 tablespoons freshly minced parsley

Salt and pepper to taste

## cooking instructions

Heat the oil in a saucepan over high heat. Add the onion and sauté until translucent. Add the carrot, celery, potatoes, stock, and bring to a boil. Reduce heat and simmer for 15 minutes. Mash the potato with a fork and continue to reduce until you obtain a creamy texture. Add the corn, milk, fish, parsley, and bring to a boil. Continue to simmer for another 5 minutes. Adjust seasoning and serve immediately.

# French Onion Soup

serves 4

## ingredients

2 tablespoons grapeseed oil
3 large onions, thinly sliced
(about 1½ pounds)
2 tablespoons Cognac (optional)
2 tablespoons flour
6 to 7 cups beef stock (low-fat and
low-sodium)

¾ cup Swiss cheese or Gruyère,
shredded (about 6 ounces)
Salt and pepper to taste

## cooking instructions

Heat the oil in a large pan over medium heat. Add the onions and cook until golden brown. Stir occasionally to avoid burning. This will take up to 20 minutes. Carefully add the cognac and flambé (optional). Sprinkle with the flour and mix well. Add the beef stock and bring to a boil over high heat. Reduce heat and simmer for 20 to 25 minutes. Skim any foam or fat that may rise to the surface. Adjust seasonings and serve immediately with the cheese.

# Oyster Stew

serves 4

## ingredients

2 cups low-fat milk
½ tablespoon olive oil
½ quart oysters
1 tablespoon parsley
Salt and pepper to taste
Cornstarch mixed with a little water

## cooking instructions

Scald the milk in a saucepan over medium heat. Thicken with a little cornstarch to obtain a sauce consistency. Carefully open the oysters and transfer their liquid to a bowl. Remove flesh and add to a pan. Add the olive oil and quickly sauté under medium heat. Add the liquid and simmer (do not boil) until the edges begin to curl. Add the hot milk, parsley, and season to taste. Bring to a simmer (do not boil) and serve immediately.

# Pumpkin Soup

serves 6

✔ *The pumpkin seeds may be browned in the oven under the broiler for a stronger flavor.*

## ingredients

1 (3 pound) pumpkin
1 teaspoon olive oil
2 large onions, sliced
(about 1 pound)
1 garlic clove, minced (optional)
6 cups chicken stock
(low-fat and low-sodium)
2 cups low-fat milk
2 fresh sage leaves

3 tablespoons low-fat Greek
yogurt
2 tablespoons pumpkin seeds
Salt and pepper to taste

## cooking instructions

Peel the pumpkin and cut the flesh into medium cubes.

Heat the oil in a large pan over high heat. Add the onions and sauté until translucent. Add the pumpkin, garlic, stock, milk, and sage, and bring to a boil. Reduce heat, cover, and simmer for 30 minutes. Transfer to a blender and puree with enough of the liquid to obtain a creamy consistency. Return to the pan, then season with salt and pepper. Before serving, add the yogurt and garnish with the pumpkin seeds.

# Soups & Salads

## Hyperthyroidism

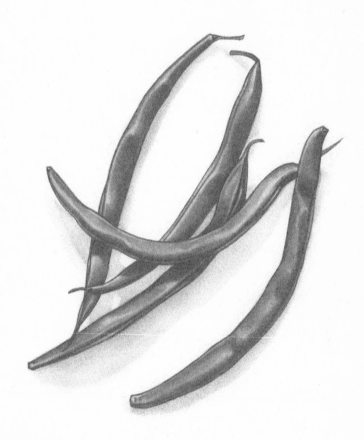

# Artichoke and Fava Bean Salad

serves 4

> ✔ *If fava beans are unavailable, use butter beans, broad beans, Windsor beans, or lima beans.*

## ingredients

*For the vinaigrette:*
2 shallots, minced
1 large garlic clove, minced
1 teaspoon Dijon mustard
4 tablespoons balsamic vinegar
6 tablespoons olive oil
2 tablespoons flaxseed oil (or olive oil, if flaxseed oil unavailable)
3 tablespoons salad herbs
Salt and pepper to taste

*For the salad:*
4 ounces Boston lettuce
8 ounces cooked fava beans
1 cup cooked artichoke hearts
8 cherry tomatoes
4 ounces feta cheese, cut into 1-inch cubes
4 teaspoons slivered almonds

## cooking instructions

*For the vinaigrette:* In a bowl, mix the shallots, garlic, mustard, and vinegar. Slowly whisk in the oils. Add the herbs and season with salt and pepper.

*For the salad:* Line a serving platter with the lettuce. Spread the fava beans, artichokes hearts, and tomatoes on top of the lettuce. Drizzle with the vinaigrette. Add the feta cheese and almonds, and serve immediately.

# Beets with Walnuts

serves 8

✔ *Suitable for Hyperthyroidism and Hypothyroidism*

## ingredients

*For the salad:*
2 large beets (about 20 ounces)
¼ cup walnuts, chopped

*For the dressing:*
1 small shallot, minced
1 large garlic clove, minced
(optional)
1 teaspoon Dijon mustard

1½ tablespoons lemon juice
1 tablespoon minced fresh
parsley
3 tablespoons walnut oil
Salt and pepper to taste

## cooking instructions

*For the salad:* Place the beets in a large pan, cover with water, and bring to a boil over high heat. Reduce heat, cover, and simmer for 30 minutes or until cooked through. Drain and cool. Peel, slice, and place in a serving bowl.

*For the dressing:* In a bowl, mix the shallot, garlic, mustard, lemon juice, and parsley. Blend in the oil and season with salt and pepper.

Mix the beets with the dressing, sprinkle the walnuts over, and serve immediately.

# Four Bean Salad

serves 6

> ✔ *This salad may be served with lettuce, tomato, and avocado.*
>
> *You may substitute one 15-ounce can of beans for each of the dried beans. Rinse canned beans before use.*

## ingredients

*For the dressing:*
1 large garlic clove, minced
2 tablespoons olive oil
4 tablespoons apple cider vinegar
2 tablespoons freshly minced salad herbs
Salt and pepper to taste

*For the salad:*
4 ounces dried garbanzo beans
4 ounces dried black beans
4 ounces dried red beans
4 ounces green beans
¼ small red onion, diced (about 1 ounce)
Salt

## cooking instructions

*For the dressing:* In a bowl, mix the garlic, oil, vinegar, and salad herbs, and season with salt and pepper.

*For the salad:* Cook the garbanzo, black, and red beans separately, following package instructions. (Generally, it takes 30 to 45 minutes to cook them.)

Cover the green beans with water in a pan, add a little salt, and bring to boil over high heat. Cook to desired tenderness. Drain and place immediately in ice-cold water to stop the cooking process. Drain and pat dry. In a large bowl, place all the beans and red onion, add the dressing, and adjust seasonings. Refrigerate for an hour before serving.

# Leeks with Walnut Vinaigrette

serves 4

## ingredients

*For the salad:*
8 small leeks

*For the vinaigrette:*
1 large garlic clove, minced
1 large shallot, minced
¼ cup walnuts, finely chopped
1 teaspoon Dijon mustard

2 tablespoons tarragon vinegar
4 tablespoons walnut oil
2 tablespoons olive oil
1 tablespoon minced fresh chives
1 tablespoon minced fresh parsley
Salt and pepper to taste

## cooking instructions

*For the vinaigrette:* In a bowl mix the garlic, shallot, walnuts, mustard, and vinegar. Slowly whisk in the oils. Add the chives and parsley, and season with salt and pepper.

*For the leeks:* Wash and trim the leeks. Place them in a pan, cover with water, and bring to a boil over high heat. Reduce heat, cover, and simmer for 10 minutes or until cooked through.

Drain and cut the leeks in half lengthwise. Mix the leeks with the vinaigrette and let cool. Refrigerate and serve cold.

# Tomato and Basil Salad

**serves 4**

## ingredients

6 to 8 fresh basil leaves

6 large tomatoes (about 2 pounds)

1 shallot, minced

1 large garlic clove, minced

2 tablespoons balsamic vinegar (preferably aged)

3 tablespoons olive oil

1 tablespoon flaxseed oil (or olive oil, if flaxseed oil unavailable)

1 tablespoon minced fresh parsley

Salt

## cooking instructions

Mince half the basil leaves and shred the remaining half.

Cut off each end of the tomatoes and discard. Slice the tomatoes and spread them on a plate. Sprinkle them with a little salt and set aside for 20 minutes.

In a bowl, mix the shallot, garlic, vinegar, and whisk in the oils. Add the minced basil and parsley, and season with salt and pepper.

Transfer the tomatoes to serving platter. Sprinkle the shredded basil, pour over the dressing, and serve immediately.

# Black Bean Soup

serves 4

## ingredients

12 ounces dried black beans, rinsed

2 teaspoons canola oil

1 large onion, finely diced (about 8 ounces)

2 large celery stalks, finely diced (about 4 ounces)

1 large carrot, finely diced (about 4 ounces)

2 garlic cloves, minced

6 cups chicken stock or vegetable stock (low-fat and low-sodium)

1 bouquet garni

Salt and pepper to taste

## cooking instructions

Place the beans in a large pot and cover with water (water should go at least 2 inches above the surface of the beans). Bring to a boil over high heat. Remove from heat and let soak 1 hour. Drain and set aside.

Heat the oil in a large pan over high heat. Add the onion and sauté until translucent. Add the celery, carrot, and garlic, and cook for 2 minutes. Add the beans, stock, and bouquet garni, and bring to a boil. Reduce heat, cover, and simmer for 45 minutes or until beans are tender. Skim off any foam forming at the liquid's surface. Remove ⅓ cup of the bean and mash with a fork. Mix the puree back into the soup. Remove the bouquet garni and season with salt and pepper. If the soup is too thick, adjust with stock. If the soup is too thin, reduce the liquid some more. Serve immediately.

# Chickpea, Tomato, and Rice Soup

serves 4

✔ *You may vary the flavor by using different herbs such as Mediterranean, Italian, or herbes de Provence.*

## ingredients

1 teaspoon olive oil
1 small onion, diced
(about 4 ounces)
3 garlic cloves, minced
1 (8 ounce) can chopped Italian
plum tomatoes
½ teaspoon freshly minced rosemary

½ cup brown rice
5 cups gluten-free chicken or
vegetable stock (low-fat and low-
sodium)
12 ounces cooked chickpeas
2 tablespoons freshly minced
parsley
Salt and pepper to taste

## cooking instructions

Heat the oil in a large pan over high heat. Add the onion and sauté until translucent. Add the garlic, tomatoes, and rosemary, and cook until the juices are evaporated. Add the rice and stock, and bring to boil. Reduce heat, cover, and simmer for 25 minutes. Add the chickpeas and continue to cook for 5 minutes or until the rice is cooked through. Add the parsley, season with salt and pepper, and serve immediately.

# Gazpacho

serves 6

## ingredients

2 slices white bread
¼ cup olive oil
3½ large tomatoes, chopped
(about 1¼ pounds)
1 medium cucumber, chopped
(about 8 ounces)
1 small onion, chopped (about 4
ounces)
1 small red or orange bell pepper,
seeded, ribs removed, and chopped
(about 3 ounces)
3 garlic cloves, chopped

1 cup tomato juice
2 tablespoons red wine vinegar
2 tablespoons chopped fresh basil
1 tablespoon freshly chopped
tarragon
Dash ground cumin
Dash Tabasco® sauce
½ lemon, juiced
Cayenne pepper
Salt to taste

## cooking instructions

Soak the bread by submerging it in cold water for 5 minutes. In a blender, puree the ingredients, except salt and cayenne pepper until smooth. Add salt and cayenne pepper. Refrigerate until cold, then serve.

# Lentil Soup

serves 4

## ingredients

2 teaspoons canola oil
1 large onion, finely diced
(about 8 ounces)
1 large carrot, finely diced
(about 4 ounces)
2 large celery stalks, finely diced
(about 4 ounces)
2 garlic cloves, minced
6 cups chicken stock
(low-fat and low-sodium)

1 small ham bone (optional)
3 cups lentils, rinsed
(about 12 ounces)
1 bouquet garni
Salt and pepper to taste

✔ *If the soup turns out too thick, adjust with stock. If the soup is too thin, reduce the liquid after passing the ingredients through a sieve. Chicken stock may be substituted with vegetable stock. You may add 8 ounces of cooked ground turkey.*

## cooking instructions

Heat the oil in a large pan over high heat. Add the onion and sauté until translucent. Add the carrot, celery, and garlic, and cook for 2 minutes. Add the stock, ham bone, if using, lentils, and bouquet garni, and bring to a boil. Reduce heat, cover, and simmer for 35 minutes. Skim the surface to remove foam as needed. Continue to simmer uncovered for 10 minutes to thicken the soup. Remove any fat that may rise to the surface of the soup. Remove the ham bone and bouquet garni. Season with salt and pepper, and serve immediately.

# Onion Soup

serves 6

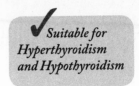

✔ Suitable for Hyperthyroidism and Hypothyroidism

## ingredients

2 tablespoons grapeseed oil
3 large onions, thinly sliced (about 1½ pounds)
2 tablespoons Cognac (optional)
2 tablespoons flour
6 to 7 cups beef stock (low-fat and low-sodium)
Salt and pepper to taste

## cooking instructions

Heat the oil in a large pan over medium heat. Add the onions and cook until golden brown. Stir occasionally to avoid burning. This will take up to 20 minutes. Carefully add the Cognac, if using, and flambé. When the flame dies, sprinkle the flour and mix well. Add the beef stock and bring to a boil over high heat. Reduce heat and simmer for 20 to 25 minutes. Skim any foam or fat that forms. Season with salt and pepper and serve immediately.

# Fish & Seafood Entrées

## Hypothyroidism

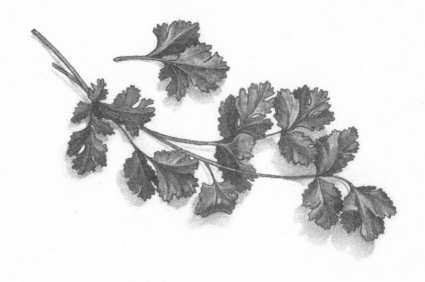

# Broiled Salmon with Dill

serves 4

## ingredients

4 (5 ounce) salmon fillets
1 tablespoon olive oil
4 to 5 fresh dill branches, minced
Salt and pepper to taste

## cooking instructions

Preheat the broiler. Rub some of the oil over the flesh side of the fillets. Lightly season with salt and pepper and spread the dill over. Place the fillets on a greased baking pan skin side up. Brush the remaining oil over the skin and broil for 3 to 4 minutes. Turn over and continue to broil for a few minutes or until the flesh starts to flake.

# Broiled Salmon with Orange Salsa

serves 4

## ingredients

1½ tablespoons grapeseed oil
4 (5 ounce) salmon fillets
2 mangos, diced
(about 14 ounces)
1 orange, diced (about 6 ounces)
1 small red onion, diced
(about 2 ounces)

2 green jalapeños, diced
1 bunch cilantro, chopped
¼ cup orange juice
Salt and pepper to taste

## cooking instructions

Mix the mangos, orange, red onion, jalapenos, cilantro and orange juice in a bowl. Season to taste and refrigerate at least 30 minutes before use.

Preheat the broiler. Brush oil over the fillets and season lightly. Broil the fish for 5 minutes on the non-skin side first. Turnover, brush more oil, and continue to cook for 5 minutes or until the flesh starts to flake. Serve immediately with the salsa.

# Honey Glazed Salmon

✓ *Serve with Vegetables Gratin (see page 101).*

serves 4

## ingredients

4 (5 ounce) salmon fillets
2 tablespoons Dijon mustard
4 teaspoons honey
2 teaspoons freshly minced thyme
1 lime
Salt and pepper to taste

## cooking instructions

Place the salmon fillets in a microwave safe dish.

In a bowl, mix the mustard, honey, thyme, and season to taste. Spread the mixture evenly over the salmon fillets. Sprinkle with a little lime juice and cover with a microwaveable top or loosely with plastic wrap. Microwave on high for 3 to 4 minutes. Time may vary based on the thickness of your fillets. Remove from the microwave and let stand for 2 minutes before serving.

# Broiled Tuna with Tarragon Sauce

serves 4

> ✓ *The cream can be substituted with Greek low-fat yogurt. If wine is not desired, substitute with stock. Serve with brown rice.*

## ingredients

1 tablespoon olive oil
1 small shallot, minced
1 garlic clove, minced (optional)
½ cup white wine
(Sauvignon Blanc)
¾ cup gluten-free vegetable stock
(low-fat and low-sodium)
8 fresh tarragon branches,
(4 branches minced, 4 whole)

2 tablespoons Dijon mustard
1 tablespoon cornstarch, mixed
with a little water
4 (5 ounce) tuna fillets
Oil spray
2 tablespoons cream (optional)
Salt and pepper to taste

## cooking instructions

Preheat the broiler. Heat the oil in a pan over high heat. Add the shallot and garlic, and sauté for 1 minute. Add the wine, stock, and half of the minced tarragon, and boil for 3 minutes. Strain and return liquid to the pan, discarding solids. Add the mustard and mix briefly. Add the cornstarch mixture, a little at a time, until the desired consistency is obtained. Remove from heat and set aside.

Place the fillets on a greased cookie sheet. Rub the whole tarragon branches on both sides of the fillets. Spray a little oil over the fillets and lightly season with pepper.

Broil for 4 to 5 minutes. Turn over and spray with a little more oil. Continue to broil until the flesh starts to flake. Remove the fillets and keep warm on a plate covered with aluminum foil. Reheat the prepared sauce, add the cream, if using, and the remaining minced tarragon, and bring to a boil. Season with salt and pepper and pour over the fillets. Serve immediately.

# Quick Tuna Daube

**serves 4**

## ingredients

*For the marinade:*
3 ounces olive oil
1 lemon, juiced
Pinch pepper

*For the fish:*
4 (5 ounce) tuna fillets
4 small canned anchovy fillets,
drained and patted dry

½ cup wild rice
4 large tomatoes
1 teaspoon olive oil
1 large onion, diced
(about 8 ounces)
3 garlic cloves (optional)
1 bouquet garni
1 cup Chardonnay (or other wine
with citrus and butter tones)
Salt and pepper to taste

## cooking instructions

*For the marinade:* Mix the oil, lemon juice, and pepper in a bowl.

*For the fish:* Make two small incisions in the top and bottom of each tuna fillet. Place one anchovy fillet in each incision. Place the tuna fillets in a plastic bag. Add the marinade and seal. Mix carefully and refrigerate for at least one hour.

Meanwhile, cook the rice according to package instructions. Make a small X incision at the top and bottom of the tomatoes. Blanch the tomatoes for 20 seconds. Remove and place in ice-cold water to stop the cooking process. Peel, seed, and dice the tomatoes. Set aside. Preheat the oven to 350°F. Remove the fish from the bag and pat dry with paper towels. Heat the oil in a nonstick pan over high heat. Add the tuna the pan, and brown for two to three minutes. Turn over and sauté for two minutes more. Remove the fillets from the pan and place on a platter. Cover with aluminum foil to keep warm. Deglaze the pan with a bit of water (see page 63 for tips on deglazing). If you prefer a less fishy smell to your dish, once deglazed disregard liquid. Add the onions and brown slightly. Add the tomatoes, garlic, bouquet garni, and wine, and bring to a boil. Transfer half of the prepared vegetables mixture to a greased casserole. Add the fish and top with the remaining vegetables mixture. Cover and bake for 20 to 25 minutes.

Remove the fish and place on a serving platter. Cover with aluminum foil to keep warm. Remove the bouquet garni. Thicken the sauce by simmering over medium heat. Season with salt and pepper and pour over the tuna fillets. Serve immediately with the wild rice.

# Tuna with Balsamic Vinegar

serves 4

## ingredients

*For the fish:*
1 cup pearl onions
2 tablespoons olive oil
1½ cups balsamic vinegar
1 shallot, minced
1 large garlic clove, minced
(optional)
1 tablespoon honey

4 (5 ounce) tuna fillets
2 tablespoons minced fresh
parsley
Salt and pepper to taste

## cooking instructions

Preheat the broiler.

Blanch the onions in boiling water for 2 minutes. Drain, cool, and peel.

Heat 1 tablespoon of the oil in a skillet over medium heat. Add the onions and brown for two to three minutes. Add the vinegar, shallot, garlic, and honey, and reduce by half.

Meanwhile, place the fillets on a greased baking pan. Brush a little of the remaining oil over the fish and lightly season with salt and pepper. Broil for 3 to 4 minutes. Turn over, drizzle the remaining oil, and continue to cook for a few minutes or until the flesh starts to flake.

Transfer the fish to a serving platter and top with the prepared onions.

# Trout Greek Style

serves 4

## ingredients

¼ teaspoon dried thyme
¼ teaspoon dried coriander
¼ teaspoon dried marjoram
¼ teaspoon dried rosemary
¼ teaspoon dried basil
4 (5 ounce) whole trout

1 tablespoon olive oil
4 teaspoons minced fresh parsley
4 teaspoons minced fresh mint
1 lemon, juiced
Salt and pepper to taste

## cooking instructions

Preheat the broiler.

*For the fish:* In a bowl blend the dried herbs. Place the trout on a flat surface and open their cavities. Sprinkle some salt, pepper, and a large pinch of the dried herbs in each trout. Add 1 teaspoon fresh parsley and 1 teaspoon fresh mint. Sprinkle lemon juice and close the trout. Place the trout on a greased baking pan. Drizzle the oil over the trout. Broil for 3 to 4 minutes. Carefully turn over, brush with oil, and continue to broil for another 3 to 4 minutes.

# Trout with Horseradish

✓ *This recipe goes well with Green Beans with Tomatoes (see page 96).*

serves 4

## ingredients

4 (5 ounce) whole trout
1 tablespoon olive oil
3 tablespoons minced fresh parsley
4 tablespoons prepared horseradish sauce (store bought)
Salt and pepper to taste

## cooking instructions

Preheat the broiler.

Clean the fish and pat dry. Sprinkle the inside of each trout with a little salt, pepper, oil, and parsley. Place the trout on a greased baking pan. Rub a little oil over the skin. Broil for 3 to 4 minutes. Carefully turn over, brush with oil, and continue to broil for another 3 to 4 minutes. Serve immediately with the prepared horseradish sauce.

# Mackerel with Steamed Vegetables

**serves 4**

## ingredients

*For the fish:*
4 (5 ounce) mackerels
1 large garlic clove, peeled
2 tablespoons olive oil
Salt and pepper

*For the vegetables:*
4 large carrots, sliced
(about 1 pound)
3 large zucchini, sliced
(about 1 pound)
1 lemon, quartered
Salt and pepper to taste

## cooking instructions

*For the fish:* Pre-heat the oven to 400°F. Sprinkle pepper and a little salt inside the mackerels. Cut the garlic clove in half and brush each half all over the bottom of a baking pan. Sprinkle half of the oil over the bottom of the pan and add the mackerel. Spread the remaining oil over the fish and bake for 20 to 25 minutes.

*For the vegetables:* Preheat a steamer. Add the carrots and cook for 4 minutes. Add the zucchini and continue to cook for 2 to 3 minutes or until desired tenderness. Transfer to a serving platter and season to taste. Serve the mackerels with the vegetables and lemon wedges.

# Italian-Style Monkfish

serves 4

## ingredients

6 large tomatoes (about 2 pounds)
½ cup brown rice
1 tablespoon olive oil
4 (5 ounce) monkfish fillets
1 large onion, sliced
(about 8 ounces)
2 tablespoons minced garlic
(optional)
1 large green bell pepper, seeded,
ribs removed, and sliced
(about 8 ounces)

1 large yellow bell pepper, seeded,
ribs removed, and sliced (about
8 ounces)
2 pinches Italian herbs
1 bunch fresh basil, shredded
Salt and pepper to taste

✔ *To deglaze: Add a liquid—such as wine, stock, or water—and swirl to dissolve cooked particles on the bottom and side of the pan. It is an important step in order to include all the extracted flavors resulting in a more flavorful sauce.*

## cooking instructions

Make a small X incision at the top and bottom of the tomatoes. Blanch the tomatoes for 20 seconds. Remove and place in ice-cold water to stop the cooking process. Peel, seed, and slice the tomatoes. Cook the rice according to package instructions. Heat the oil in a large nonstick pan over high heat. Lightly season the fish with salt and pepper, add to the pan, and brown for two to three minutes. Turn over and sauté for 2 minutes more. Remove the fish and set aside on a plate. Deglaze the pan with a little water (see above for tips on deglazing). Add the onions and cook for 2 minutes. Add the garlic, tomatoes, bell peppers, and Italian herbs, and sauté for 2 minutes. Slide the fillets back into the pan, cover, and cook for 20 minutes over low heat. Remove the fillets and place on a serving platter. Cover with aluminum foil to keep warm. Mix the basil into the vegetables and season with salt and pepper. Pour over the fish and serve immediately with the rice.

# Scallops with Tangerines

serves 4

## ingredients

6 tangerines
1 cup orange juice
1 teaspoon minced ginger
3 teaspoons olive oil, plus more for drizzling
1 pound scallops

1 shallot, minced
8 ounces mushrooms
2 tablespoons minced fresh parsley
Salt and pepper

## cooking instructions

Peel and segment the tangerines. Place the orange juice and half of the ginger in a saucepan and bring to a boil over high heat. Reduce to ¼ cup and set aside.

Heat 1 teaspoon oil in a saucepan over high heat. Add the mushrooms, shallot, and remaining ginger, and sauté briefly. Add parsley and lightly season with salt and pepper. Heat the remaining 2 teaspoons oil in a large saucepan over high heat. Lightly season the scallops, add to the pan, and sear for 1½ minutes. Turn over and sear for 1½ minutes more. Add the tangerine segments, reduced orange juice, and continue to sauté for 1 minute. Serve immediately with the mushrooms and drizzle a little oil.

# Sea Bass with Ginger and Lime

serves 4

## ingredients

*For the fish:*
1 tablespoon olive oil
4 (5 ounce) sea bass fillets
½ cup lime juice
½ small onion, diced
(about 2 ounces)
1 teaspoon minced garlic
(optional)
1 tablespoon minced fresh ginger
½ cup Chardonnay wine (or other
wine with lemon-lime tones)
1 tablespoon honey

1 teaspoon fresh rosemary
Cornstarch mixed with a little
water
2 tablespoons minced fresh
parsley
Salt and pepper to taste

*For the vegetables:*
1 pound carrots
1 pound green beans
1 lime, juiced
Salt and pepper to taste

## cooking instructions

*For the vegetables:* Steam vegetables until desired tenderness. Mix with lemon juice, season with sea salt and pepper, and set aside.

*For the fish:* Heat the oil in a nonstick pan over medium heat. Lightly season the fillets with salt and pepper, add to the pan, and brown for two to three minutes. Turn over and cook for 2 minutes more. Add about ⅓ of the lime juice, cover, and reduce heat. Cook the fillets until the flesh starts to flake. Remove the fish from the pan and place on a serving platter. Cover with aluminum foil to keep warm. Add the onions, garlic, ginger, wine, remaining lime juice, honey, and rosemary to the pan. Mix well and bring to a boil. Reduce the sauce to ⅔ cup. Add a little of the cornstarch mixture and bring to a boil to thicken. Strain, discarding solids, and return to pan. Add the parsley and adjust seasoning. Pour over the fillets and serve immediately with the cooked vegetables.

# Shrimp Scampi

serves 4

## ingredients

*For the pasta:*
½ cup whole wheat pasta

*For the shrimp:*
4 tablespoons olive oil
2 garlic cloves, minced (optional)
2 pounds large shrimp, shelled
and deveined

2 red bell peppers, seeded, ribs
removed, and sliced
(about 1 pound)
½ lemon, zest removed and juiced
2 tablespoons minced fresh
parsley
Salt and pepper to taste

## cooking instructions

*For the pasta:* Cook according to package directions.

*For the shrimp:* Heat the oil and garlic in a large pan over medium heat. Add the shrimp and cook for 1 minute stirring occasionally. Add the bell peppers, lemon zest and juice, parsley, and season with salt and pepper. Continue to cook for two minutes or until the shrimp is cooked through stirring occasionally. Add the cooked pasta, toss, and serve immediately.

# Meat, Poultry & Vegetarian Entrées

## Hypothyroidism

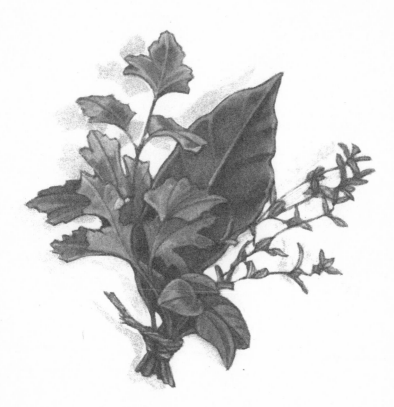

# Chicken Breast with Dijon Mustard

✔ *Suitable for Hyperthyroidism and Hypothyroidism*

serves 4

## ingredients

4 (5 ounce) skinless chicken breasts
Canola oil
1 tablespoon Dijon mustard
2 teaspoons lemon juice
½ teaspoon garlic powder (optional)
Salt and pepper to taste

## cooking instructions

Preheat the oven to 375°F. Place the chicken breasts in a lightly oiled pan. In a bowl, mix the mustard, lemon juice, and garlic powder. Spread over the chicken breasts and season to taste. Bake for 20 to 25 minutes, or until cooked through. Time may vary depending on the thickness of the breasts.

# Herbed Chicken

serves 4

✓ *Suitable for Hyperthyroidism and Hypothyroidism*

## ingredients

4 teaspoons olive oil
4 tablespoons dried Italian herbs
4 (6 ounce) bone-in,
skin-on chicken breasts

1 large lemon, cut in 8 slices
Pepper to taste

## cooking instructions

Preheat the oven to 375°F. Mix the olive oil, Italian herbs, and season with pepper. With your fingers, carefully separate the chicken skin slightly from the flesh, being careful not to break the skin. Spread the herbed oil mixture over the chicken flesh, add 2 lemon slices per breast, and push back the skin. Place the breasts in a baking dish and bake for 20 to 25 minutes, or until cooked through. Time may vary depending on the thickness of the breasts. Serve immediately and remember to discard the skin when eating.

# Roasted Chicken Breast with Sweet Potatoes

✓ *Suitable for Hyperthyroidism and Hypothyroidism*

**serves 4**

## ingredients

2 tablespoons olive oil
4 (4 ounce) skinless
chicken breasts
4 sweet potatoes, unpeeled and
quartered (about 1 pound)
1 large yellow bell pepper, seeded,
ribs removed, and chopped
(about 8 ounces)

1 large zucchini, chopped
(about 8 ounces)
1 teaspoon dried Italian herbs
Salt and pepper to taste

## cooking instructions

Preheat the oven to 400°F.

In large bowl mix 1 tablespoon oil with the chicken and transfer to a roasting pan. Toss the remaining 1 tablespoon oil with the sweet potatoes, bell pepper, and zucchini. Transfer to the roasting pan arranging them around the chicken breasts. Sprinkle the Italian herbs and lightly season with pepper. Roast until the chicken and vegetables are tender, 25 to 30 minutes, turning halfway through the cooking time. Remove from the oven, season lightly with salt, and serve immediately.

# Chicken Burgers with Lettuce Wraps

serves 4

## ingredients

2 white anchovy fillets
4 tablespoons garlic Caesar
Litehouse Foods dressing
4 (4 ounce) organic
chicken burgers
2 tablespoons olive oil

4 garlic cloves, minced
(optional)
16 lettuce leaves
4 tablespoons Parmesan cheese
Canola oil
Salt and pepper to taste

## cooking instructions

In a food processor, puree the anchovy fillets with the dressing. Add a little water to thin out. Lightly season the burgers with salt and pepper and shape them to fit in the lettuce leaves. Do not allow the meat to touch the leaves. Heat up the olive oil with the garlic. Remove at first boil and set aside.

Preheat the grill to medium-high heat. Grease the grill with canola oil before adding the burgers. Cook them for 3 to 5 minutes on each side or until cooked through. Meanwhile, carefully brush the garlic oil over the lettuce leaves.

Place two leaves on a plate, top with one burger, spread 1 tablespoon of the dressing, sprinkle 1 tablespoon cheese, and fold any lettuce overhang over the top. Top with 2 more leaves and tuck underneath to seal. Repeat with the remaining ingredients. Serve immediately with your favorite sides. Use toothpick to hold the lettuce in place if necessary

# New York Steak with Mushrooms and Onions

serves 4

## ingredients

4 (4 ounce) New York steaks
5 teaspoons olive oil
1 pound onions, sliced (about 2 large onions)
1 pound mushrooms, sliced
2 garlic cloves, minced (optional)
2 tablespoons freshly minced parsley
¼ cup Dijon mustard
Salt and pepper to taste

## cooking instructions

Preheat the broiler. Brush 1 teaspoon each of the olive oil over the steaks and season with pepper. Broil for 3 to 5 minutes on each side or to desired tenderness. Sprinkle a little salt before serving.

Meanwhile, heat the remaining 1 teaspoon olive oil in a nonstick pan over medium heat. Add the onions and brown slightly. Add the mushrooms and garlic, and continue to cook until the mushrooms are slightly tender. Add the parsley and season with salt and pepper.

Plate the vegetables in the center of a serving platter and top with the steaks. Serve with Dijon mustard on the side.

# Cornish Hen with Red Cabbage

serves 4

## ingredients

2 tablespoons grapeseed oil
2 Cornish hens
4 slices turkey bacon
1 large onion, sliced
(about 8 ounces)
2 Granny Smith apple, sliced
(about 8 ounces)
1 red cabbage, sliced
(about 1½ pounds)

4 cups chicken stock (low-fat and
low-sodium)
2 cloves
1 laurel leaf
1 teaspoon caraway seeds
Mustard
Salt and pepper to taste

## cooking instructions

Blanch the red cabbage into boiling salted water. Rinse the Cornish hen under cold water, pat dry, and lightly season.

Heat half of the oil in a sauté pan. Sear the Cornish hen on all sides (about 10 minutes).

Heat the remaining oil in a Dutch oven or brasier. Add the bacon, onion, apples, and sweat for two minutes. Add the red cabbage, stock, cloves, laurel leaf, caraway seeds, and bring to boil. Top with the Cornish hen, cover, and cook for 40 to 50 minutes in the oven. Serve with mustard on the side.

# Lamb Chops with Herbs

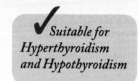

✓ *Suitable for Hyperthyroidism and Hypothyroidism*

**serves 4**

## ingredients

1 tablespoon minced garlic (optional)

1 tablespoon minced fresh parsley

4 tablespoons whole wheat bread crumbs

1 tablespoon minced fresh Italian herbs

3 tablespoons Dijon mustard

Olive oil

8 (3½ ounce) lamb loin chops (about 1¾ pounds total)

Salt and pepper to taste

## cooking instructions

Preheat the oven to 400°F.

In a bowl, combine the garlic, parsley, bread crumbs, and Italian herbs, then season with salt and pepper. Add the mustard and just enough oil to bind the mixture together.

Heat 1 teaspoon oil in a sauté pan over high heat. Add the lamb chops and brown on both sides, about three to four minutes each side.

Remove from heat. Place the chops on a greased baking pan. Spread the breadcrumb mixture over the chops and press hard. Bake for 10 minutes for medium rare or up to 15 minutes for welldone.

# Meatloaf
# with Tomato Sauce

serves 6

✓ *If buffalo meat is not available, substitute with organic sirloin ground beef.*

## ingredients

1 teaspoon olive oil
1 small onion, minced
(about 4 ounces)
1 celery stalk, minced
(about 2 ounces)
2 garlic cloves, minced (optional)
1 pound ground buffalo meat
¾ pound ground chicken
or turkey meat
3 ounces gluten-free ground oats
1 large egg, beaten

3 ounces chicken stock (low-fat
and low-sodium)
1 teaspoon salt
¼ teaspoon pepper
½ teaspoon dried Italian herbs
¼ teaspoon dry mustard
⅛ teaspoon dried sage
10 ounces diced tomato
1 cup tomato sauce

## cooking instructions

Preheat the oven to 350°F.

Heat the oil in a pan over high heat. Add the onion, celery, and garlic, and cook for 2 minutes. Transfer to a mixing bowl and add the remaining ingredients, except the tomato sauce. Mix well and place the meatloaf into a greased loaf pan. Bake for 1 hour to 1½ hours or until cooked through. Serve with your favorite tomato sauce.

# Turkey Breast with Sage Aromas

serves 4

> ✔ *Use the turkey meat to make soup, salad, sandwich, etc.*

## ingredients

2 tablespoons olive oil
1 turkey breast (about 2 pounds)
1 tablespoon ground sage
3 to 4 fresh sage leaves
½ cup chicken stock (low-fat and low-sodium)
Cornstarch
Salt and pepper to taste

## cooking instructions

Preheat the oven to 350° F.

Mix the ground sage with a little pepper and spread all over the turkey breast under its skin. Be careful not to break the skin. Brush olive oil over the skin. Place the turkey skin-side up in a roasting pan. Pour the chicken stock in the pan, add the sage leaves, and bake for an hour or until a meat thermometer registers 180° F.

Remove the turkey breast from the pan, cover with aluminum foil to keep warm. Remove the sage leaves from the sauce and thicken with a little cornstarch and water mixture. Adjust seasonings and serve over the turkey breast slices.

# Mediterranean Portobello Burger

✓ *Suitable for Hyperthyroidism and Hypothyroidism*

serves 4

## ingredients

4 teaspoons olive oil
4 large portobello mushroom caps
4 slices onion
2 garlic cloves, minced (optional)
4 tablespoons roasted red bell pepper spread
4 teaspoons chopped black olives

4 teaspoons feta cheese
8 slices tomato
8 large basil leaves
Lettuce leaves wide enough to wrap portobello mushrooms
Apple cider vinegar
Pepper to taste

## cooking instructions

Preheat the grill to medium heat.

Brush 1 teaspoon olive oil and sprinkle pepper over each portobello. Grill the mushrooms for 2 minutes on each side. Add the onion and grill. Turn the mushrooms so that the top of the mushroom cap is on the grill. Fill the underside cavity with the garlic, bell pepper spread, and olives, and season with salt and pepper. Grill for another minute or two.

Place each portobello mushroom on a few lettuce leaves (cap side down), add 1 teaspoon feta cheese, 1 grilled onion slice, 2 slices tomato, 2 basil leaves, and sprinkle vinegar. Close the lettuce leaves to seal and serve immediately.

# Meat, Poultry & Vegetarian Entrées

## Hyperthyroidism

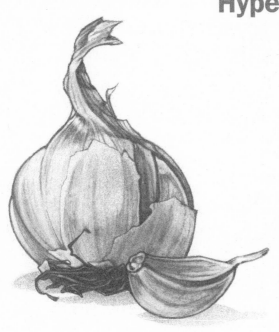

# Chicken Breast with Asian Glaze

serves 4

## ingredients

4 (5 ounce) chicken breasts with
bones and skin
2 tablespoons maple syrup
1 tablespoon green tea leaves
1 tablespoon Oriental
hot mustard

1 garlic clove, minced
2 tablespoons sesame seeds
1 teaspoon ground ginger
Canola oil
Salt and pepper to taste

## cooking instructions

Preheat the oven to 350°F. Wash and pat dry the chicken breasts. Carefully pass your fingers between the meat and the skin to loosen up the skin without breaking it.

Heat the maple syrup, tea, mustard, garlic, and ginger in a saucepan over low heat until well blended. Season to taste and set aside. Lift up the chicken skin and brush the mixture over the chicken meat. Sprinkle the sesame seeds under the skin. Brush canola oil over the skin and roast for 30 minutes, or until cooked through. Remove skin before serving.

# Chicken Breast
# with Wild Mushrooms

serves 4

## ingredients

2 teaspoons olive oil
4 (5 ounce) skinless chicken breasts
2 shallots, minced
3 garlic cloves, minced
½ cup red wine (Syrah, Shiraz, or Barbaresco)
1 cup chicken stock (low-fat and low-sodium)
2 fresh rosemary sprigs

Cornstarch mixed with a little water
1 tablespoon minced fresh parsley
Salt and pepper to taste

*For the side:*
2 teaspoons olive oil
1 pound wild mushrooms, cleaned and sliced
1 pound cooked chestnuts
1 tablespoon minced fresh parsley
Salt and pepper to taste

## cooking instructions

For the chicken: Heat the oil in a sauté pan over high heat. Lightly season the chicken with salt and pepper, add to the pan, and brown on both sides for three minutes each side. Add the shallots, garlic, wine, and reduce by half. Add ½ cup of the chicken stock and 2 sprigs rosemary, and bring to a boil. Reduce heat, cover, and simmer for 10 to 15 minutes or until the chicken is cooked through.

Remove the chicken breasts from the pan and place on a serving platter. Cover with aluminum foil to keep warm. Add the remaining ½ cup stop stock to the pan and reduce the liquids to a little less than 1 cup. Thicken with a little cornstarch mixture. Add the parsley together with, any rendered chicken juices, and bring to a boil. Adjust seasonings and pour over the chicken.

For the side: Heat oil in a nonstick pan over medium heat. Add the mushrooms and cook until almost cooked through. Add the chestnuts, mix well, season to taste, and continue to cook for 2 to 3 minutes. Add a little sauce from the chicken and mix well.

Serve the chicken breasts with the mushrooms and chestnuts.

# Lemon Chicken

serves 4

> ✓ *Suitable for*
> *Hyperthyroidism*
> *and Hypothyroidism*

## ingredients

3 tablespoons olive oil
5 lemons (4 juiced, 1 cut into wedges)
1 tablespoon freshly minced poultry herbs
4 (4 ounce) skinless chicken breasts
Pepper to taste

## cooking instructions

Mix in 2 tablespoons of the oil, the juice, and herbs, and season with pepper. Place the chicken pieces in a plastic bag. Pour the lemon marinade over the chicken and refrigerate for at least one hour rotating every 10 minutes.

Preheat the broiler. Remove the chicken breasts from the marinade and pat dry. Place them on a cookie sheet greased with a little of the remaining 1 tablespoon oil and brush the rest of the remaining oil over each breast. Broil for approximately 6 to 7 minutes on each side. Watch carefully to avoid burning. Serve immediately with the lemon wedges.

# Stuffed Chicken Breast with Boursin

serves 4

## ingredients

4 (4 ounce) chicken breasts
4 pinches dried Italian herbs
2 ounces Boursin (garlic and herbs), divided into four portions
8 fresh large basil leaves
1 tablespoon olive oil, plus more for stir-frying
1 large shallot, thinly sliced
1 cup chicken stock (low-fat and low-sodium)

Cornstarch mixed with a little water
2 tablespoons minced fresh parsley
2 pounds fresh dandelions, washed and pat dry
Salt and pepper to taste
Kitchen twine or toothpicks

## cooking instructions

Preheat the oven to 350°F. Place the chicken breasts between two plastic wrap sheets. Flatten with a mallet until fairly thin. Sprinkle pepper and a pinch of Italian herbs on each breast. Spread one portion of Boursin and 2 basil leaves, and roll each breast tightly. Secure with kitchen twine so they do not unroll. Heat the oil in an ovenproof sauté pan over high heat. Add the turkey rolls, side face down, and brown for two to three minutes. Turn over and brown two minutes more. Once browned, add the shallot and ½ cup of the chicken stock. Bring to a boil and place in the oven for 10 to 12 minutes. Remove the rolls from the pan and place on a serving platter. Cover with aluminum foil to keep warm. Add the remaining ½ cup stock to the pan (be careful, it just came out of the oven!) and reduce the sauce to a little less than 1 cup. Thicken with a little cornstarch mixture. Add the parsley and any rendered turkey juices, and bring to a boil. Adjust seasonings and pour over the turkey. Serve immediately with the steamed dandelions. While the sauce is reducing, stir-fry the dandelions until slightly wilted. Season to taste and serve with the stuffed chicken.

# Lamb Chops with Garlic Spread

serves 4

## ingredients

4 cups green beans
(about 2 pounds)
6 teaspoons olive oil
2 tablespoons minced garlic

2 teaspoons freshly minced
parsley
2 teaspoons freshly minced
rosemary
½ teaspoon dry crushed
red pepper
4 (4 ounce) loin lamb chops
Salt and pepper to taste

## cooking instructions

Trim and place the green beans in a pan. Cover with water, add 1 teaspoon of salt, and bring to boil. Reduce heat and simmer until tender. Drain and transfer to a serving bowl. Add 2 teaspoons olive oil, season with salt and pepper, and mix well.

In a bowl, mix 2 teaspoons of the remaining oil, the garlic, parsley, rosemary, and dry crushed red pepper. Rub the spread over the lamb chops.

Heat the remaining 2 teaspoons oil in a nonstick pan over medium heat. Add the lamb chops and cook for 3 to 4 minutes on each side or to desired doneness. Serve immediately with the prepared green beans.

# Pork Loin with Tomato Coulis

serves 4

## ingredients

6 large tomatoes (about 2 pounds)
1 tablespoon olive oil
4 (5 ounce) pork loin chops
3 garlic cloves, minced
2 shallots, minced
Pinch sugar
1 tablespoon flour
½ cup Chardonnay

½ cup vegetable stock (low-fat and low-sodium)
1 teaspoon tomato paste
1 fresh rosemary sprig
Cornstarch mixed with a little water
2 tablespoons minced fresh basil
2 tablespoons minced fresh parsley
Salt and pepper to taste

## cooking instructions

Make a small X incision on the top and bottom of the tomatoes. Blanch the tomatoes for 20 seconds. Place in ice-cold water to stop the cooking process. Peel, seed, and dice the tomatoes.

Heat the oil in a deep pan over high heat. Lightly season the loin chops with salt and pepper, add to the pan, and brown on both sides, about three to four minutes each side. Add the garlic, shallots, diced tomatoes, and sugar, and reduce heat to medium. Sprinkle the flour over the vegetables and mix well. Continue to cook for 2 minutes. Add the wine, stock, tomato paste, and rosemary, and bring to a boil. Cover and cook for 25 minutes over low heat.

Remove the chops and set aside in a serving platter. Cover with aluminum foil to keep warm. Remove the rosemary and puree the sauce with a hand mixer or in a blender. Reduce the sauce to concentrate its flavors. If necessary, thicken with a little cornstarch mixture. Add the basil, parsley, any rendered loins juices, and bring to a boil. Adjust seasonings and pour over the chops.

# Stuffed Turkey Breast Italian Style

✓ *Suitable for Hyperthyroidism and Hypothyroidism*

serves 4

## ingredients

4 (4 ounce) skinless turkey breasts
4 pinches dried Italian herbs
4 slices prosciutto ham
2 ounces goat cheese,
sliced in 4 pieces
8 large fresh basil leaves
1 tablespoon olive oil

1 large shallot, thinly sliced
¼ cup Madeira
1 cup chicken stock
(low-fat and low-sodium)
Cornstarch mixed with a little
water
2 tablespoons minced fresh
parsley
Salt and pepper to taste
Toothpicks or kitchen twine

## cooking instructions

Preheat the oven to 350°F.

Place the turkey breasts between two plastic wrap sheets. Flatten with a mallet until fairly thin. Lightly season with salt and pepper, and sprinkle a pinch of Italian herbs on each breast. To each breast add one slice of ham, one slice of cheese, and 2 basil leaves, and roll tightly. Secure with a few toothpicks so they do not unroll.

Heat the oil in an ovenproof sauté pan over high heat. Add the turkey rolls, folded side down, and brown, about two to three minutes. Turn over and sauté, two minutes more. Once browned, add the shallot, Madeira, ½ cup of the chicken stock. Bring to a boil and place in the oven for 10 to 12 minutes. Remove the rolls from the oven and place on a serving platter. Cover with aluminum foil to keep warm. Add the remaining ½ cup stock to the pan (be careful, it just came out of the oven!) and reduce the sauce to with a little less than 1 cup. Thicken with a little cornstarch mixture. Add the parsley and any rendered turkey juices, and bring to a boil. Adjust seasonings and pour over the turkey.

# Turkey Breast with Cherries

serves 4

## ingredients

½ cup brown rice
1 tablespoon grapeseed oil
4 turkey breasts
1 large shallot, minced
1 teaspoon black peppercorns, cracked
2 pinches dried thyme
1 bay leaf

1 cinnamon stick
1 cup pomegranate juice
1 cup brown sauce
1 cup pitted cherries
2 tablespoons minced fresh parsley
Salt and pepper to taste

## cooking instructions

Preheat the oven to 350°F.

Cook the rice according to the package instructions.

Heat the oil in an ovenproof skillet over high heat. Lightly season the turkey breasts with salt and pepper, add to the pan, and brown on both sides. Transfer to the oven and continue to cook for 10 minutes. Remove the pan from the oven with oven mitt and transfer the turkey breasts to a plate. Cover with aluminum foil to keep warm. Handling the pan with the oven mitt, discard any fat from the pan. Add the shallot, peppercorns, thyme, bay leaf, cinnamon, and pomegranate juice, and deglaze the bottom and sides of the pan (see page 63 for tips on deglazing). Bring to a boil and reduce by half. Remove the cinnamon stick. Add the brown sauce and reduce the sauce to 1 cup. Add the cherries and bring to a boil. Add the turkey breasts back to the pan with any rendered juices, and bring to a boil. Add the parsley. Bring to a simmer, adjust seasonings, and serve immediately.

# Tuscan Beef Stew

**serves 8**

## ingredients

6 teaspoons olive oil
6 ounces onion, diced
(about 1 medium onion)
2 garlic cloves, minced
2 pounds lean beef stew meat
½ cup Tuscan red wine
(or beef stock)

6 ounces celery stalks, sliced
(about 3 celery stalks)
2 whole cloves
2½ cups diced tomatoes
3 parsley branches, minced
3 medium potatoes, quartered
(about 18 ounces potatoes)
1 bouquet garni
Salt and pepper to taste

## cooking instructions

Heat 2 teaspoons of oil in a pan over high heat. Add the onion and garlic, and sauté until translucent. Transfer to a stockpot. Using the same pan, add 2 teaspoons of the remaining oil and brown half the meat. Transfer the meat to the stockpot and repeat the process with the remaining 2 teaspoons oil and beef. Deglaze the pan with the wine (or stock), swirling to dissolve the particles on the bottom and sides of the pan. Transfer the deglazing liquid to the stockpot.

Heat the stockpot over medium heat. Add the celery, cloves, tomatoes, parsley, and bouquet garni, and season with pepper. Cook over low heat for 1 hour. Add the potatoes and continue to cook for 20 minutes. If the meat is not tender enough, remove the potatoes, and continue to cook until tender. Adjust seasonings and serve immediately.

# Pasta with Vegetables and Sun-Dried Tomatoes

serves 4

## ingredients

8 ounces penne
4 teaspoons olive oil
½ small onion, diced
(about 2 ounces)
1 medium yellow bell pepper,
diced (about 6 ounces)
2 garlic cloves, minced
Florets from 1 large head
broccoli (about 8 ounces)

10 sun-dried tomatoes packed in
oil, julienned, plus some of the
packing oil
¼ teaspoon red pepper flakes
2 tablespoons pine nuts
1 bunch fresh basil leaves,
julienned
Salt and pepper to taste

## cooking instructions

Cook the pasta according to package directions. Drain and return to
the pan. Mix in 1 teaspoon of the oil.

Heat 2 teaspoons of the oil in a pan over high heat. Add the onion
and sauté until translucent. Add the bell peppers and garlic, and cook
for 2 minutes, mixing occasionally. Add the broccoli and sun-dried
tomatoes, and continue to cook until the vegetables are tender. Add a
little of the oil from the sun-dried tomatoes, the pine nuts and basil,
and season with salt and pepper. Blend in the cooked pasta and serve
immediately.

# Tofu and Collard Greens Burgers

**serves 4**

## ingredients

8 ounces tofu

6 ounces cooked collard greens

1 small onion, diced
(about 4 ounces)

1 small carrot, shredded
(about 2 ounces)

2 scallions, chopped

2 garlic cloves, minced (optional)

1⅓ cups water crackers

4 teaspoons almond butter

2 tablespoons minced salad herbs

Salt and pepper to taste

## cooking instructions

Mix all the ingredients in a food processor until well combined. Form 4 patties and grill on each side for 4 to 5 minutes. Serve immediately.

# Side Dishes & Snacks

## Hypothyroidism

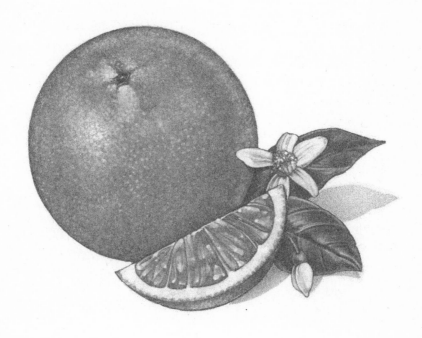

# Baby Bell Peppers with Tuna

**24 stuffed baby bell peppers**

## ingredients

12 ounces tuna canned in water

2 tablespoons minced fresh parsley

2 tablespoons minced fresh chives

¼ cup finely chopped scallions

1 lemon, juiced

6 tablespoons canola mayonnaise

24 baby bell peppers (approximately 4 cups)

Salt and pepper to taste

## cooking instructions

In a bowl, mix the tuna, parsley, chives, and scallions. Sprinkle a little bit of lemon juice. Mix in the mayonnaise and season with salt and pepper. Refrigerate until needed.

Cut off the tops of the bell peppers. Remove the seeds and ribs. Fill with the tuna mixture and serve immediately.

# Butternut Squash with Cinnamon

✔ *Suitable for Hyperthyroidism and Hypothyroidism*

**serves 4**

## ingredients

2 pounds butternut squash
1 orange (about 6 ounces)
3 tablespoons maple syrup
1 teaspoon cinnamon
1½ tablespoons grapeseed oil
Salt and pepper to taste

## cooking instructions

Preheat the oven to 350°F.

Remove two large zest strips from the orange. Mince and set aside. Juice the orange and set aside.

Halve the squash lengthwise and remove the seeds and strings. Rub the inside with grapeseed oil and season to taste. Place on a greased cookie sheet, skin side down, and bake for 35 to 40 minutes or until tender.

Meanwhile heat the orange juice, maple syrup, and cinnamon in a pan over high heat. Reduce by half.

Remove the squash from the oven, scoop out the flesh, and transfer to a food processor. Add the orange zest, 1 tablespoon of the concentrated juice, and purée. Add more concentrated juice as needed to reach the desired thickness. Adjust seasonings and serve immediately.

# Provence-Style Tomatoes

serves 4

## ingredients

4 large tomatoes
6 teaspoons olive oil
1 bunch fresh basil leaves, minced
¼ cup wheat breadcrumbs
Salt and pepper to taste

## cooking instructions

Preheat the oven to 375°F.

Cut the tomatoes in half. Lightly season with salt and pepper and sprinkle ¼ teaspoon oil over each tomato half. Add some basil and 1 teaspoon breadcrumbs over each half. Place in a baking dish. Sprinkle remaining oil over the breadcrumbs. Bake for 20 to 25 minutes and serve immediately.

# French Macaroni and Cheese

serves 6

✓ *Healthy variation for kids: Mix in diced vegetables, cooked white meat, salmon, or tuna.*

## ingredients

8 ounces whole wheat macaroni
2 tablespoons unsalted butter
4 ounces Gruyère cheese, finely shredded
¼ cup 2% low-fat milk, heated
Pinch nutmeg
Salt and pepper to taste

## cooking instructions

Cook the macaroni according to package directions. Drain and return to the pan. Over very low heat, mix in the butter, Gruyère, and milk. Continue to mix until the cheese is melted. Remove from heat and add a pinch of nutmeg. Season with salt and pepper, and serve immediately.

*Gruyère cheese is what makes this dish so unique. However, if not available, you may substitute Swiss cheese.*

# Green Beans with Tomatoes

**serves 4**

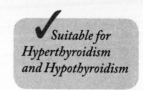

*✓ Suitable for Hyperthyroidism and Hypothyroidism*

## ingredients

1 pound green beans, ends trimmed

1½ tablespoons olive oil

½ cup pearl onions, peeled and halved

2 garlic cloves, minced (optional)

1 cup cherry tomatoes

2 pinches minced fresh thyme

2 tablespoons minced fresh basil

1 tablespoon minced fresh parsley

Pepper to taste

## cooking instructions

Bring to a boil enough water to cover the green beans. Add 1 teaspoon of salt. Add the green beans and bring to a boil. Reduce heat and simmer until cooked through. Drain and set aside.

Heat 1 tablespoon of the oil in a sauté pan over medium heat. Add the pearl onions and sauté until golden brown. Add the garlic and cook for 1 minute. Add the green beans, tomatoes, and herbs, and cook until the vegetables are warmed through. Blend in the remaining oil, season with salt and pepper, and serve immediately.

# Stuffed Mushrooms with Tapenade

24 mushrooms

✔ *You can also just fill raw mushroom caps with the prepared tapenade and serve.*

*The tapenade may be refrigerated up to 5 days. Cover the tapenade with a thin layer of olive oil to avoid dryness.*

## ingredients

24 large mushrooms,
stems removed
1 cup pitted black olives
1 ounce capers, drained, rinsed,
and patted dry
2 ounces anchovy fillets
2 garlic cloves, minced (optional)

3 ounces olive oil
1 bunch fresh parsley, minced
1 teaspoon lemon juice

## cooking instructions

Preheat the broiler. Empty and clean the center of each mushroom caps. Place the mushrooms on a baking sheet. Broil for 3 to 4 minutes until the mushrooms start to sweat. Do not overcook, as the mushrooms will start to shrink. Remove from the oven and set aside to cool.

In a food processor, puree the olives, capers, anchovies, garlic, oil, and lemon juice. Add pepper to taste. Fill each mushroom cap with the tapenade, sprinkle with parsley, and serve immediately.

# Salmon Bruschetta

**24 bruschetta**

## ingredients

1⅓ cups fresh basil
⅔ cup fresh parsley
2 tablespoons minced
fresh lemon thyme
½ cup walnuts
2 garlic cloves (optional)
1 lemon, zested and juiced
¼ cup olive oil

1 country bread loaf
24 smoked salmon slices, rolled
(about 1 pound, 2 ounces)
Salt and pepper to taste

## cooking instructions

In a food processor, puree the basil, parsley, lemon thyme, walnuts, garlic, 1 tablespoon lemon zest, and 1 tablespoon lemon juice. Gradually add the oil until you have a smooth paste. Season with salt and pepper. If too thick, add a little more oil.

Preheat the broiler. With a serrated knife, cut the walnut bread into ½-inch-thick slices. Cut each slice in half. Place the slices on a baking sheet. Broil on both sides until golden brown. Cool before using.

Spread some paste over each bread slice. Add one salmon roll, sprinkle each with a little lemon juice, and serve immediately.

# Sugar Snap Peas with Salmon

serves 4

## ingredients

1 tablespoon olive oil
2 cups sugar snap peas
2 garlic cloves, minced (optional)
1 lemon
4 ounces salmon, thinly sliced
Salt and pepper to taste

## cooking instructions

Remove strings along both lengths of the sugar snap peas. Heat a
wok with the olive oil over medium heat. Add the garlic and sauté
quickly. Add the sugar snap peas and sauté until almost tender.
Add the salmon and sauté quickly. Sprinkle with lemon juice,
season to taste, and serve immediately.

# Stuffed Eggplant

serves 4

## ingredients

1 egg
½ cup wheat breadcrumbs
½ teaspoon dried Italian herbs, minced
2 medium eggplants
(about 1 pound)
Olive oil

1 medium onion, diced
(about 6 ounces)
1 tablespoon minced garlic
(optional)
4 basil leaves, minced
¼ cup minced fresh parsley
Salt and pepper to taste

## cooking instructions

Place the egg in a saucepan and cover with water. Bring to a boil over medium heat and cook for 10 minutes. Drain and cool in cold water. Peel the egg and mash with a fork in a bowl.   Meanwhile, mix the breadcrumbs and dried Italian herbs.

Preheat the oven to 425°F. Cut the eggplants in half and remove the flesh without damaging the skin. Make very small incisions on the rim tops to allow the skin to stretch a bit, this will prevent breakage during cooking. Place the eggplant halves in a small greased baking pan and brush them with oil. Set aside. In a food processor puree the eggplant flesh and mashed egg. Heat 1 teaspoon oil in a nonstick pan over medium heat. Add the onions and garlic, and sauté for 2 minutes. Add the eggplant mixture and fresh herbs, and cook for 2 minutes more. Season with salt and pepper and fill the eggplant cavities with this mixture. Sprinkle the herbed breadcrumbs over the eggplant halves and sprinkle with a little olive oil. Bake for 30 to 35 minutes.

# Vegetables Gratin

**serves 4**

## ingredients

1 large yellow squash, chopped large (about 8 ounces)

1 large red bell pepper; seeded, ribs removed, and chopped large (about 8 ounces)

1 large green bell pepper; seeded, ribs removed, and chopped large (about 8 ounces)

1 large zucchini, chopped large (about 8 ounces)

1 large onion, quartered (about 8 ounces)

2 medium sweet potatoes, chopped large (about 8 ounces)

2 garlic cloves, minced (optional)

2 tablespoons lemon juice

2 tablespoons olive oil

1 fresh thyme branch, minced

2 tablespoons freshly minced parsley

2 tablespoons grated Parmesan cheese

Salt and pepper to taste

## cooking instructions

Cut the vegetables the same size for even cooking.

In a bowl mix the garlic, lemon juice, thyme, parsley, and season to taste. Mix in the remaining vegetables (except sweet potatoes) and set aside for at least an hour.

Preheat the oven to 425°F. Place the sweet potatoes in a roasting pan. Mix in half of the olive oil, sprinkle with pepper, and bake for 20 minutes. Sprinkle the remaining oil over the potatoes. Add the prepared vegetables with the marinade and continue to bake for 20 minutes. Sprinkle the cheese, brown under the broiler, and serve immediately.

# Side Dishes & Snacks

## Hyperthyroidism

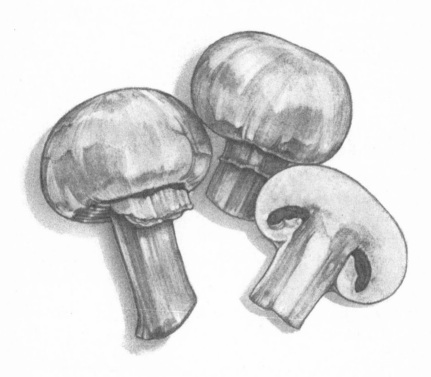

# Rice with Lentils

serves 8

## ingredients

2½ cups lentils, rinsed
2 teaspoons olive oil
2 large onions, diced
(about 1 pound)
2 teaspoons minced garlic
1 teaspoon ground cumin
1 teaspoon ground coriander

1 teaspoon paprika
2 tablespoons minced fresh
parsley
1⅓ cups long-grain rice, rinsed
Salt and pepper to taste

## cooking instructions

Place the lentils in a pan and add enough water to cover them. Bring to a boil over high heat and simmer for 10 minutes. Drain and set aside.

Heat the oil in a large pan over high heat. Add the onions and sauté until translucent. Add the garlic, lentils, cumin, coriander, paprika, and parsley, and season with salt and pepper. Add 6 cups water. Bring to a boil, reduce heat, cover, and simmer for 10 minutes. Add the rice and bring to a boil. Reduce heat, cover, and cook for 20 minutes or until tender. Adjust seasonings and remove from heat. Set aside covered for 5 minutes before serving.

# Wild Rice with Vegetables

serves 8

## ingredients

1⅓ cups wild rice
2 teaspoons olive oil
2 medium onions, finely diced
(about 12 ounces)
2 medium carrots, finely diced
(about 6 ounces)
3 large celery stalks, finely diced
(about 6 ounces)

1 garlic clove, minced
4 cups vegetables stock
2 tablespoons minced fresh
parsley
Salt and pepper to taste

## cooking instructions

Rinse the rice well and drain. Heat the oil in a deep pan over high heat.
Add the onions, carrots, celery, and garlic, and sauté for 2 minutes. Add
the rice and sauté for 1 minute. Add the stock and parsley, and bring
to a boil. Cover, reduce heat, and cook until tender (approximately 45
minutes but it may depend of the type of rice you use. For best results,
see package instructions). Season with salt and pepper and remove from
heat. If necessary, strain and serve immediately.

# Roasted Pumpkin

serves 4

> ✓ You can also use the cooked pumpkin to make a purée or soup. Thin out with low-fat milk until the necessary consistency is reached. You can also use the cooked pumpkin as a base for dips or as a dessert base.

## ingredients

3 pounds sugar pumpkin
1 tablespoon grapeseed oil
Pumpkin pie spice mix
Salt and pepper to taste

## cooking instructions

Cut open the pumpkin, remove seeds and clean the inside with a spoon. Brush oil inside the cavity, season to taste, and place opening side down on a baking sheet. Roast for 30 to 45 minutes or until tender. Cut out and sprinkle with a little pumpkin pie spices before serving.

# Orange-Glazed Carrots

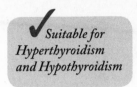
✓ *Suitable for Hyperthyroidism and Hypothyroidism*

serves 4

## ingredients

1 tablespoon grapeseed oil
1 small sweet onion, diced (about
4 ounces)
6 cups baby carrots
(about 1½ pounds)
1 teaspoon honey

1½ cups orange juice
3 tablespoons minced fresh
parsley
Salt and pepper to taste

## cooking instructions

Heat the oil in a saucepan over high heat. Add the onions and
carrots, and brown slightly. Add the honey and just enough orange
juice to cover the vegetables (about 1½ cups). Bring to a boil
and cook over medium heat until the liquid is almost completely
evaporated. Add the chopped parsley and season lightly with salt
and pepper.

# Eggplant Mediterranean Style

serves 4

✓ *If ground thyme and oregano are difficult to find, use fresh versions and mince as small as possible.*

## ingredients

2 small eggplants, both ends trimmed (about 1 pound)
1 tablespoon paprika
1 tablespoon ground ginger
1 tablespoon garlic powder
1 teaspoon coriander
1 teaspoon cumin

½ teaspoon cayenne pepper
¼ teaspoon ground thyme
¼ teaspoon ground oregano
2 tablespoons olive oil
Salt

## cooking instructions

Cut eggplant slices lengthwise and arrange on baking sheet. Mix all the spices together. On both sides of the eggplant slices, brush olive oil, season with salt, and sprinkle the prepared spices. Preheat the broiler or barbecue. Broil or grill until golden brown, about 2 minutes per side.

# Porcini Mushrooms Provence Style

serves 4

## ingredients

2 pounds Porcini mushrooms
3 tablespoons olive oil
2 tablespoons minced garlic
½ teaspoon minced fresh thyme
2 tablespoons minced fresh parsley
1 tablespoon minced fresh basil
Salt and pepper to taste

## cooking instructions

Clean the porcini by brushing off the dirt and then wiping them carefully with a damp cloth. Slice the mushrooms and set aside.

Heat the oil in a large nonstick pan over medium heat. Add the garlic and cook for 15 seconds. Add the mushrooms, thyme, and sauté for 2 to 3 minutes. Add the parsley and basil, and season with salt and pepper. Cook for 2 minutes more and serve immediately.

# Potato Parsnip Puree

serves 8

## ingredients

8 medium potatoes
(about 3 pounds)
1 large parsnip (about 6 ounces)
3 large garlic cloves, peeled
½ cup vegetable stock

1 tablespoon olive oil
1 tablespoon minced fresh parsley
1 tablespoon minced fresh chives
Salt and pepper to taste

## cooking instructions

Peel and quarter the potatoes and parsnip. Place them in a deep pan and add enough cold water to cover. Add the garlic cloves, ¼ teaspoon salt, and bring to a boil over high heat. Cook until cooked through, about 20 to 25 minutes. Strain through a sieve, reserving the cooking liquid, and puree with a potato masher. Add the vegetable stock and oil, and mix briefly. If too thick, add a little of the reserved cooking liquid to get to the right consistency. Mix in the parsley and chives, season with salt and pepper, and serve immediately.

# Spinach with Pine Nuts and Raisins

serves 4

## ingredients

2 tablespoons grapeseed oil
⅓ cup plump raisins
1 tablespoon pine nuts
2 pounds fresh spinach, washed and patted dry
Salt and pepper to taste

## cooking instructions

Heat the oil in a nonstick pan over medium heat. Add the raisins, pine nuts, and sauté for 1 minute. Add the spinach and sauté very briefly. Season with salt and pepper and serve immediately. The spinach should be barely wilted to avoid turning to mush.

# Broccoli and Pistachio Vinaigrette

serves 4

> ✓ *You may substitute 2 tablespoons balsamic vinegar for the lemon juice.*

## ingredients

1 teaspoon Dijon mustard
1 tablespoon minced shallots
1 teaspoon minced garlic
4 tablespoons olive oil
3 tablespoons lemon juice
1 tablespoon minced fresh parsley

Florets from 2½ large heads broccoli (about 1½ pounds)
4 teaspoons chopped pistachios
Salt and pepper to taste

## cooking instructions

In a bowl, mix the mustard, shallot, garlic, oil, lemon juice, and parsley, and season with salt and pepper.

Preheat a steamer. Add the broccoli and cook for 2 to 3 minutes or to desired doneness. Heat the vinaigrette in a pan over medium heat until warm. Transfer the cooked broccoli to a bowl. Pour the warmed vinaigrette and toss. Sprinkle the pistachios and serve immediately.

# Olive Paste and Red Bell Pepper Bruschetta

24 bruschetta

> ✔ *You may use this olive paste on sandwiches, in salads, or with vegetable snacks. It may be refrigerated for up to 5 days. Cover the paste with a thin layer of olive oil to avoid dryness.*

## ingredients

2 large red bell peppers (about one pound)
1½ cups pitted black olives
2 ounces capers, rinsed and pat-dried
4 large garlic cloves, minced
½ lemon, juiced
½ cup olive oil

2 ounces anchovy fillets, rinsed and pat-dried
1 French baguette
Salt and pepper to taste

## cooking instructions

Preheat the broiler. Place the red bell peppers on a baking sheet and char on all sides. If you have a gas stovetop, you may char the bell peppers over the flames. Once blackened on all sides, place in a paper bag and seal. Let stand for 10 minutes. Peel and seed the bell peppers. Remove ribs and slice into ½-inch wide strips.

In a food processor, puree the olives, capers, garlic, oil, lemon juice, and anchovy fillets. The paste should be smooth and spreadable. If it is too thick, add a little more olive oil. Season with salt and pepper and refrigerate for 30 minutes.

With a serrated knife, cut the baguette into ¾-inch-thick slices. Place the slices on a baking sheet. Broil on both sides until golden brown. Cool before use.

Spread some olive paste on each bread slice and top with 1 slice of red bell-pepper. Serve immediately.

# Desserts

## Hypothyroidism

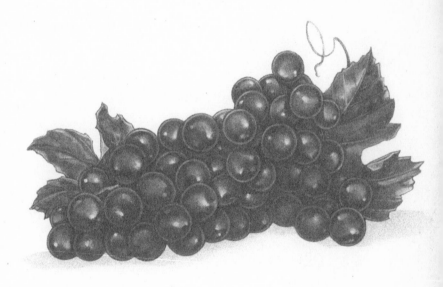

# French Crêpes

**serves 10**

## ingredients

1 cup whole wheat flour
2 extra-large eggs
1 tablespoon sugar
2 tablespoons unsalted butter, melted

2 tablespoons vanilla extract
Pinch salt
1 cup milk
Grapeseed oil

## cooking instructions

Place the flour in a bowl. Blend in the eggs, sugar, butter, vanilla, and salt. Slowly, whisk in the milk. Let the batter rest for 30 minutes. Before use, add a little water to thin out the batter (you should aim for a thinner consistency than pancakes).

Heat a nonstick pan or crêpe pan over medium heat. Soak a small piece of paper towel with 1 teaspoon grapeseed oil and swirl quickly over the pan. Add enough batter and swirl to cover the entire bottom. Cook until golden brown and turn over. Cook until slightly golden brown. Add filling (see pages 117-118) or remove from pan and set aside for later use.

# Apple Filling for Crêpes

**serves 10**

## ingredients

5 large apples
¼ cup lemon juice
½ cup plus 2 tablespoons apple butter
¼ cup plus 1 tablespoon walnuts
¼ cup plus 1 tablespoon raisins
10 crêpes (see page 116)
Cinnamon to taste

## cooking instructions

Peel and slice the apples. Place them immediately in lemon juice to prevent browning. Poach the apples in the lemon juice plus enough water to cover them halfway (heightwise) and a little cinnamon. Cook until the apples are just barely tender. Remove from heat, drain, and set aside.

Spread 1 tablespoon apple butter on a warm crêpe. Add 2 ounces apples in the center. Sprinkle 1½ teaspoons walnuts, 1½ teaspoons raisins, and cinnamon. Fold each side over the center and continue to cook for a minute. Repeat with remaining crêpes. Serve immediately.

# Strawberry Filling for Crêpes

serves 10

## ingredients

10 tablespoons blackcurrant or boysenberry preserves
1⅓ pounds strawberries, trimmed and thinly sliced
10 crêpes (see page 116)

## cooking instructions

Spread 1 tablespoon preserves evenly on a warm crêpe. Add 2 ounces
strawberries in the center. Fold each side over the center and continue
to cook for a minute. Repeat with remaining crêpes. Serve immediately.

# Cherry Compote
# with Vanilla Ice Cream

serves 4

## ingredients

1 pound English or
Montmorency cherries
3 ounces sugar
½ cup water
¼ teaspoon almond extract

¼ teaspoon arrowroot or cornstarch mixed with a little water
2 cups low-fat vanilla ice cream

## cooking instructions

Remove cherry pits and stalks. Place the cherries in a pan, add the water, sugar, almond extract, and bring to a boil over medium heat. Simmer for 10 minutes. Thicken with the arrowroot mixture and remove from heat. Cool and refrigerate. Divide among four bowls and top with the ice cream.

# Chocolate Cake with Raspberry Coulis

✔ *You may serve with extra raspberries on the side.*

serves 12

## ingredients

*For the cake:*
6 large eggs, seperated
½ cup plus 1 tablespoon sugar
8 ounces bittersweet chocolate, chopped
½ cup unsalted butter
2 tablespoons raspberry liquor

*For the coulis:*
2 cups fresh raspberries
1 teaspoon lemon juice
¼ cup maple syrup

## cooking instructions

*For the cake:* Preheat the oven to 350°F. Grease the bottom and sides of 9-inch cake pan. Line the bottom with parchment paper.

In a mixer, whisk the egg yolks with the ½ cup sugar until pale in color and set aside. In a double boiler, melt the chocolate and butter over low heat. Mix until well incorporated. Remove from the double boiler, blend in the raspberry liquor, and let cool a bit. Add the chocolate mixture to the egg yolks mixture and mix well. Whip the egg whites until soft peaks form. Add the 1 tablespoon sugar and continue to beat until the stiff peaks form. Carefully fold in one-third of the egg whites into the cake batter. Fold in another one-third and then the final one-third. Do not overmix, as the egg whites may collapse and your cake will be flat and heavy.

Carefully pour the batter into the prepared pan and bake for 30 minutes or until a tooth pick inserted in the center comes out dry. Transfer to a cooling rack and let cool for 10 minutes. Remove pan and discard the parchment paper. Let cool completely.

*For the coulis:* In a blender, mix the raspberries. Add the juice and maple syrup. Mix until smooth, and thin out with a little water, if necessary. Pass through a sieve to remove seeds. Refrigerate and serve cold, on the side, with the chocolate cake.

# Orange Salad with Champagne

serves 8

✔ *Suitable for Hyperthyroidism and Hypothyroidism*

✔ *For a colorful touch, try adding a few pomegranate seeds to the finished dish.*

## ingredients

8 large oranges
3 tablespoons orange blossoms honey
1 teaspoon coriander seeds (optional)
1½ cups water
1 cup dry Champagne
2 tablespoons Grand Marnier® or orange liqueur

## cooking instructions

Peel and slice the oranges using a paring knife. Do not leave any white membranes on the oranges, as they have a bitter taste.

Heat the honey, coriander, if using, and water in a saucepan over high heat for approximately 10 minutes to end up with 1 cup. Strain into a large bowl and set aside to cool. Mix in the Champagne and liqueur. Add the orange slices and refrigerate at least an hour before serving.

# Marie's Oatmeal Cookies

**20 cookies**

## ingredients

7 ounces almond meal
¾ cup brown sugar
1½ teaspoons baking powder
¾ teaspoon baking soda
¼ teaspoon salt

1 extra large egg
2 ounces apricot preserves
1 cup Old Fashioned
Quaker® Oats
2 ounces unsalted butter

## cooking instructions

Preheat the oven to 350°F. Prepare a couple of cookie sheets covered with a silpat mat or parchment paper. Mix the almond meal, brown sugar, baking powder, baking soda, and salt. Blend in the egg and the preserves. Melt the butter and let cool for a minute. Add the oats to the almond mixture and mix well. Add the melted butter. Scoop out the dough with a #30 scoop (about 1 ounce cookie) onto the cookie sheet, placing the mounds 3 inches apart to allow for spreading. Refrigerate for 30 minutes. Flatten the dough slightly with your palm and bake for 12 minutes or until golden brown. Let cool in the pan before transferring to a cooling rack.

This type of cookie will be moist. Don't store for more than 2 days at room temperature. It absorbs moisture quickly and can become very soggy. The best way to store them would be to freeze immediately after they cool down. Defrost at room temperature as needed or quickly defrost in the microwave for 5 to 7 seconds.

You may add ½ cup of raisins, dried fruits, coconut, chocolate chips, chopped dates, nuts, or a combination of various ingredients. Remember, any of these ingredients will add calories to the original recipe.

You may also add 1 teaspoon cinnamon and/or ½ teaspoon allspice.

**Marie's Chocolate Oatmeal Cookies:** Reduce almond meal to 6 ounces and add ⅓ cup pure cocoa powder. Follow the same direction as recipe above. Add the cocoa powder with the oats.

# Pomegranate and Strawberry Parfait

serves 2

✔ Option: Add 1 tablespoon of ground flaxseeds per serving.

## ingredients

1½ cups strawberries
2 ounces pure acai, no sugar added
1 teaspoon vanilla extract
1 cup low-fat Greek yogurt
2 tablespoons pomegranate seeds

## cooking instructions

Mix the strawberries with vanilla extract and acai. Marinade for 30 minutes. Spoon half the fruit mixture into four parfait glasses. Top with yogurt and finish with the berries. Sprinkle with the pomegranate seeds and serve immediately.

# Strawberries with Spicy Red Wine

serves 4

✔ *Suitable for Hyperthyroidism and Hypothyroidism*

## ingredients

4 teaspoons walnuts
4 large apples
9 teaspoons pomegranate preserves
4 tablespoons pomegranate juice
4 tablespoons pomegranate seeds

## cooking instructions

In a saucepan, combine the wine, honey, vanilla, peels, and peppercorns. Bring to a boil over high heat. Continue to boil until the wine is reduced by half. Remove from heat and strain, discarding the solids.

Place the strawberries in a bowl and pour the hot wine over. Mix well and let cool. Refrigerate for at least 2 hours. Serve cold.

# Yogurt with Prunes

**serves 4**

## ingredients

1 pound prunes
3 ounces sugar
12 ounces water
16 ounces low-fat Greek yogurt

## cooking instructions

Soak the prunes in water for two hours. Transfer to a pan,  add
the sugar, and bring to a simmer over medium heat. Reduce heat
and continue to cook for 1 hour. Remove from heat and let cool.
Refrigerate until cold.

Divide the yogurt into four serving bowls, top with the prunes, and
serve immediately.

# Desserts

## Hyperthyroidism

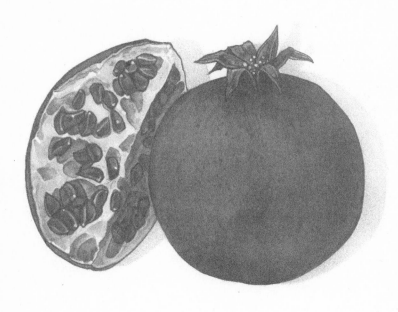

# Apple and Pear Minestrone

serves 2

## ingredients

1 medium apple, brunoise
(about 5 ounces)
1 medium pear, brunoise
(about 5 ounces)
¾ cup jasmine green tea
(or your favorite)
1½ teaspoons honey

½ teaspoon pumpkin pie spices
1 small ginger root, minced
½ teaspoon lemon zest
½ teaspoon grapeseed oil

## cooking instructions

Heat the oil in a deep saucepan over high heat. Add the apple and sauté for two minutes. Add the pear, spices, ginger, lemon zest, and sauté another minute. Add the green tea and bring to a boil. Remove from heat and transfer to a serving bowl. Cool at room temperature. Refrigerate for an hour or, even better, overnight to allow flavors to emerge. Serve cold.

# Baked Apples with Pomegranate Preserves

serves 4

## ingredients

4 teaspoons walnuts
4 large apples
9 teaspoons pomegranate preserves
4 tablespoons pomegranate juice
4 tablespoons pomegranate seeds

## cooking instructions

Preheat the broiler. Cover the bottom of a baking sheet with parchment paper. Add the walnuts and broil until slightly browned. Remove from the sheet, cool, and chop.

Preheat the oven to 400°F.

Wash and core the apples, being careful not to break through the bottom of the apples. Place them in a baking pan that is just the right size to keep the apples close to each other. Put 1 teaspoon of pomegranate preserves in the cavity of each apple. Pour 1 tablespoon of pomegranate juice into the cavity of each apple. Add a little hot water to the pan (about ¼ inch high). Cover the pan with aluminum foil and bake for 20 minutes. Remove foil and baste with the pan liquids. Continue baking uncovered for 4 to 5 minutes. If necessary, add a little more water to avoid burning.

Place each apple in a serving dish. Scrape particles from the pan and transfer the liquid to a saucepan. Blend the liquid with the remaining pomegranate preserves and bring to boil over high heat. Pour over the apples, sprinkle the walnuts, pomegranate seeds, and serve immediately.

# Baked Apples with Toasted Walnuts

serves 4

## ingredients

4 teaspoons walnuts
4 apples
9 teaspoons orange preserves
4 tablespoons Chardonnay (with apple and citrus tones)

## cooking instructions

Preheat the broiler. Cover the bottom of a baking sheet with parchment paper. Add the walnuts and toast until slightly browned. Remove the walnuts from the sheet, cool, and chop.

Lower the oven to 400°F. Wash and core the apples, being careful not to break through the bottom of the apples. Place them in a baking pan that is just the right size to keep the apples close to each other. Put 1 teaspoon of preserves in the cavity of each apple. Pour one tablespoon of wine over the cavity of each apple. Add a little hot water in the pan, about ¼ inch high. Then cover the pan with aluminum foil and bake for 20 minutes. Remove cover and baste with the liquid in the pan. Continue baking uncovered for 4 to 5 minutes. If necessary, add a little more water.

Place each apple in a dessert dish. Scrape particles from the pan and transfer along with the remaining liquids to a saucepan. Blend the liquid with the remaining 5 teaspoons preserves and bring to a boil over high heat. Pour over the apples, sprinkle the walnuts, and serve immediately.

# Dates with Almonds

serves 4

✔ *You may also store each portion in a plastic bag for a healthy prepared snack.*

## ingredients

8 dates
4 tablespoons almonds

## cooking instructions

Divide the dates and almonds in 4 dessert plates and serve immediately.

# Fruit Juice Popsicles

serves 2

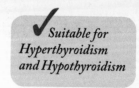

✓ *Suitable for Hyperthyroidism and Hypothyroidism*

## ingredients

¾ cup pomegranate juice
½ cup orange juice
4 ounces acai, no sugar added

## cooking instructions

Mix the juices in a blender. Transfer to popsicle molds and freeze.

# Melon Soup

serves 4

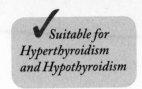 ✓ *Suitable for Hyperthyroidism and Hypothyroidism*

## ingredients

2 cantaloupes (about 4 cups flesh)
2 tablespoons honey
(warmed in the microwave for about 10 seconds)
4 mint leaves
1 lemon, juiced

## cooking instructions

Cut the cantaloupes in half. Remove all the seeds. Spoon out the flesh and place in a blender. Add the honey, mint, and lemon juice. Puree and refrigerate. Serve cold.

# Papaya Brulée

**serves 2**

## ingredients

2 small papayas
4 teaspoons brown sugar

## cooking instructions

Preheat the broiler. Cut the papayas in half and remove the seeds. Spread the sugar over each half. Place under the broiler and grill until caramelized. This is pretty quick, so keep an eye on the papayas. It will take approximately

1 minute.

# Peach with Apricot Coulis

serves 4

## ingredients

4 peaches
12 apricots
1 tablespoon honey
1 teaspoon lemon juice
1 rosemary branch
4 teaspoons almonds

## cooking instructions

Cut apricots in half and remove pits. Place the apricots in a pan. Add
½ cup water, honey, rosemary, lemon juice, and bring to a boil. Reduce
heat, cover, and simmer for ten minutes. Purée in a blender and transfer
to a serving bowl. Let cool and refrigerate. Peel and cut the peaches
in half. Place the peach halves in a serving platter, drizzle with some
apricot sauce and the almonds. Serve with the remaining apricot sauce
on the side.

# Poached Pears with Black Muscat

serves4

## ingredients

½ lemon
½ orange
2 large ripe Bosc pears
12 ounces black Muscat
1 cinnamon stick
1 teaspoon vanilla extract
1 teaspoon ground cardamom
1½ tablespoons honey

## cooking instructions

Remove a large piece of lemon peel from the lemon and set aside. Juice the lemon and set aside. Remove a large piece of orange peel from the orange and set aside. Juice the orange and set aside.

Peel, halve, and core the pears. Place them in a bowl and add the reserved lemon juice. Mix well to prevent browning.

In a saucepan, combine the wine, peels, orange juice, cinnamon stick, vanilla, honey, and cardamom. Bring to a simmer over medium heat. Add the pears with the lemon juice, and simmer until tender when pierced with a knife, 25 to 30 minutes. Remove the pears and set aside in a serving bowl. Reduce the wine until it thickens like syrup to concentrate the flavors. Cool slightly, pass through a sieve, and add the sauce to the pears. Refrigerate and serve cold.

# Winter Fruit Salad

serves 4

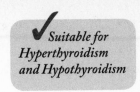
✓ *Suitable for Hyperthyroidism and Hypothyroidism*

## ingredients

1 small banana, sliced
6 ounces berries or mango
1 apple, diced
6 ounces grapes
1 orange, peeled and segmented
¼ cup pomegranate seeds
2 tablespoons lemon juice

## cooking instructions

Blend all the fruits in a large bowl. Mix in the lemon juice, pomegranate seeds, and refrigerate until use.

# References

## Online Resources:

**American Thyroid Association**
www.thyroid.org

**Everyday Health**
www.everydayhealth.com

**Health Square**
www.healthsquare.com

**The Herb Companion**
www.herbcompanion.com

**LIVESTRONG**
www.livestrong.com

**Mayo Clinic**
www.mayoclinic.com

**Medline Plus®**
www.nlm.nih.gov/medlineplus/

**WebMD**
www.webmd.com

**The World's Healthiest Foods**
www.whfoods.com